Review us on Amazon

★★★★★

Scan me

-OR-

Touch or Click here to review

Table Of Contents

Day #

Day

Day

Day

Day

Disclaimer:

The recipes in this book are provided for educational and inspirational purposes only. They are not intended as medical advice. Before starting any new diet or nutrition plan – especially one that replaces meals – consult your physician or a qualified healthcare provider to ensure it's right for your individual needs.

Dedication

To every woman, rediscovering her strength, one sip at a time. You've given endlessly — to family, to work, to others. This time, it's your turn.

Thank you!

Page intentionally left blank

Introduction: Why Your Body Deserves a Reset

"You've spent decades caring for everyone else. These 21 days are for you."

There comes a time in every woman's life — often somewhere after forty — when the mirror starts reflecting more than just a face. It shows fatigue, stress, and the quiet signs of being last on your own list.

If you've ever felt that your body isn't responding the way it used to… that your energy dips by mid-afternoon… that bloating, cravings, or restless nights have become your "new normal" — you're not alone.

We live in a world that runs on convenience, caffeine, and comparison. Our bodies have become the casualty of busyness. Smoothie Queen™ was born out of the realization that health doesn't have to be complicated — it has to be consistent.

This 21-Day Full Body Detox isn't about starving, restricting, or punishing yourself. It's about coming home to your body — giving it real nutrients, real rest, and real love again.
For the next three weeks, you'll do something revolutionary: You'll simplify. You'll slow down. You'll nourish yourself — not because you have to, but because you deserve to.

Nourishment, Not Deprivation

Imagine waking up feeling lighter. Your skin glowing. Your digestion calm. Your mind clear.

That's what happens when you stop fighting your body and start feeding it what it actually craves — balance. These 21 days are your permission slip to reset, recharge, and reclaim your rhythm.

Welcome to Smoothie Queen™ — where healing tastes delicious. 🖤

🍎 *How the 21-Day Detox Works*

This program is refreshingly simple — one smoothie replaces one meal each day.

No calorie counting, no guilt, no confusion. Just 21 days of pure, whole-food goodness that gives your body a break from heavy, processed meals and reawakens your natural energy. Each recipe has been crafted to help you:

- ■ Detox gently and naturally
- ■ Balance hormones and reduce bloating
- ■ Support digestion and skin clarity
- ■ Rebuild steady energy and focus
- ■ Feel in control of your health again

Combine creativity & nutrition 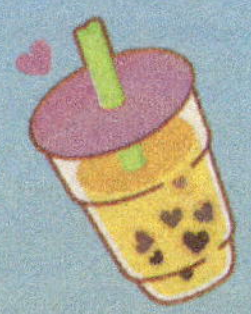

You'll notice how your cravings shift.

Your digestion steadies.

And your body begins to thank you in the language of calm and vitality.

The Ritual That Changes Everything!

Every day, you'll:

1. Blend your daily smoothie — replace one meal (rotating between breakfast, lunch, and early dinner).
2. Reflect for 5 quiet minutes, pay attention to smoothie illustration and note how you feel.
3. Scan the QR code — watch the recipe on www.SmoothieQueen.blog to see how your smoothie should look and learn small tips from real creators.

This simple ritual turns healthy living into something joyful and mindful.

By combining creativity with nutrition, you'll form habits that stick — because they're fun, visual, and rewarding.

Designed simply for your lifestyle

Your Detox Toolkit

Success begins with preparation — and this plan gives you all the tools to make your reset seamless.

Blender Tips

- Use a high-speed blender for smooth texture and maximum nutrient extraction.
- Start with liquid first, greens second, frozen fruit last.

Don't be afraid to experiment — smoothies are forgiving

Keep these on hand for your 21-day journey:

- Base Liquids: almond milk, coconut water, oat milk, or filtered water
- Greens: spinach, kale, cucumber, celery
- Fruits: bananas, berries, mango, pineapple, apples
- Boosters: chia, flaxseed, oats, protein powder, nut butters
- Extras: honey, cinnamon, cocoa powder, collagen peptides

Substitution Guide

- No banana? Try mango or avocado.
- No almond milk? Use oat or coconut milk.
- Dairy-free? Use plant-based yogurt or skip entirely.

This detox is flexible — it's designed to work with your lifestyle, not against it.

Rejuvinate, Refresh, Rekindle

⬛ 21-Day Checklist & Progress Tracker

⬛ Drink one smoothie daily (replace one meal).

⬛ Stay hydrated — aim for 8 glasses of water per day.

⬛ Move your body — even 15 minutes counts.

⬛ Record your sleep, mood, and energy levels.

- By Day 7, you'll feel lighter.
- By Day 14, you'll feel clearer.
- By Day 21, you'll feel like yourself again.

❤ Listen to Your Body

This is your journey — not a race.

- If you need to rest, rest.
- If you crave something warm, add a soup or light salad.

This isn't punishment. It's partnership — between you and your body.

"You've taken care of everyone else long enough. Now it's time to take care of the woman who made it all possible — you."

Welcome to Smoothie Queen™ — where wellness meets joy, one smoothie at a time. Lets start. Shall we?

Day 1 : Morning Glow Starter

Breakfast : Cleanse & Bloat Relief

- ½ cucumber (peeled and chopped)
- 1 cup fresh spinach leaves
- ½ lemon (peeled)
- 5–6 fresh mint leaves
- 1 small green apple (optional, for sweetness)
- 1 cup cold water or coconut water
- Ice cubes (as desired)

- Calories: ~80
- Key Nutrients:
- Vitamin C (lemon, spinach) – boosts immune function and skin radiance
- Vitamin K (spinach, cucumber) – supports circulation and bone health
- Antioxidants (mint, apple) – help reduce inflammation
- High water content – aids hydration and gentle detoxification
- Fiber: ~3g

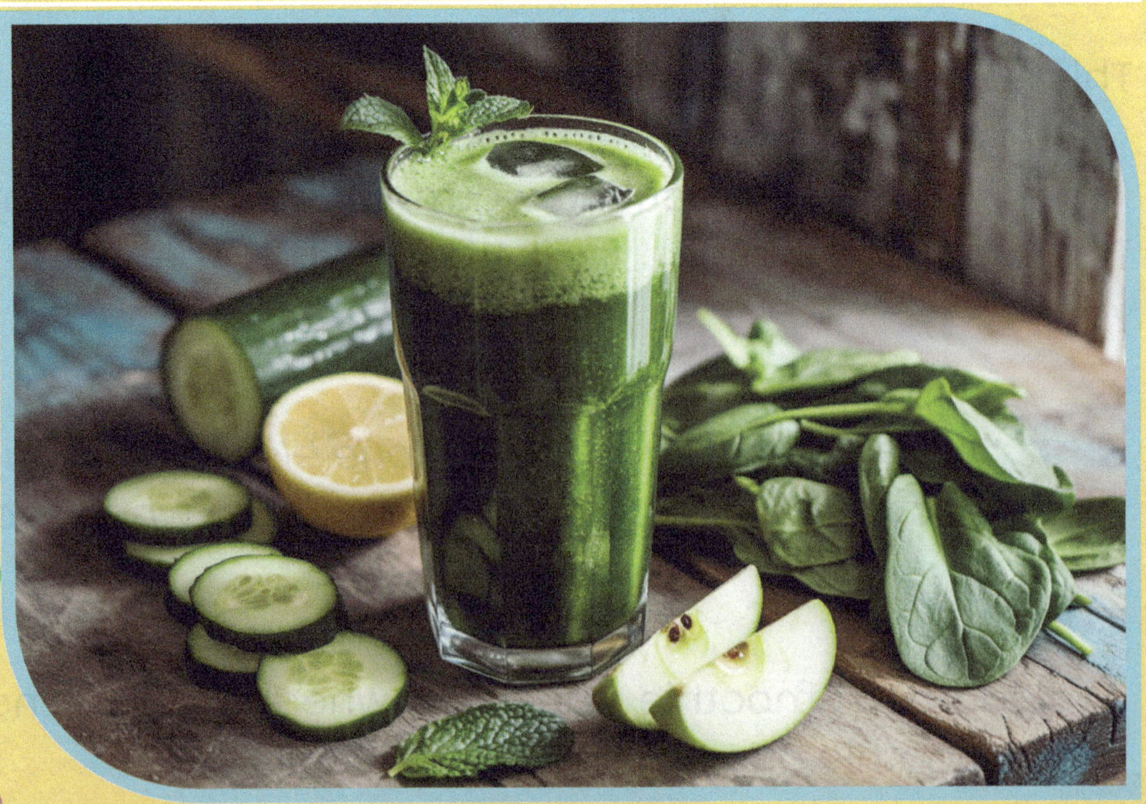

Find this recipe on our website

scan me

Nutritional & Health Benefits of Morning Glow Starter

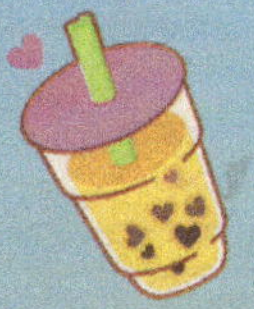

A Refreshing Beginning for Cleanse & Clarity

Your Morning Glow Starter Smoothie marks the first step of your 21-day transformation – a bright, hydrating blend that gently wakes up your body and mind.

Light, clean, and invigorating, this smoothie flushes out toxins, hydrates your cells, and sets a positive tone for the day ahead.

This is the "reset button" your system has been craving – a way to begin each morning with freshness, calm, and intention.

Ingredient Power Breakdown

Cucumber – High in water and silica, it flushes toxins and supports glowing, hydrated skin.

Spinach – Loaded with iron, folate, and antioxidants to energize your metabolism and circulation.

Lemon – A natural liver cleanser and vitamin C powerhouse that enhances collagen and immune defense.

Mint – Refreshes digestion and reduces morning bloating.

Green Apple (Optional) – Adds light sweetness while providing pectin fiber for gut health.

Coconut Water (Optional) – Delivers electrolytes for deep cellular hydration.

Why It Matters for Women Over 40

This smoothie's gentle alkalizing and detoxifying properties help:

Rebalance your body's pH for clearer skin and better digestion

Support liver health for hormone balance and natural energy

Flush excess sodium to reduce bloating and puffiness

Hydrate tissues and joints for flexibility and glow

Starting your day hydrated and alkaline helps reset your metabolism – and your mindset.

Pro Tip:

Drink this smoothie within 30 minutes of waking up. Your body absorbs nutrients best before breakfast, making this blend a perfect jumpstart to your detox journey.

Mind-Body Connection & Lifestyle Insights

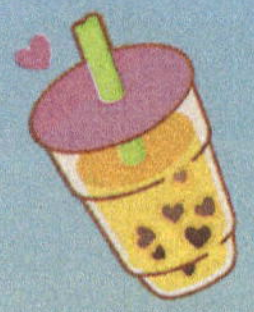

Today's Focus: Cleanse & Awaken

Every new beginning deserves stillness and intention.
As you sip your first smoothie, take a deep breath – you're not just cleansing your body, you're creating space for clarity, energy, and joy to enter your life.
This is your invitation to slow down and tune in.

Mind-Body Benefits

Rehydrates and rebalances mood after overnight fasting.
Promotes calm wakefulness instead of caffeine spikes.
The cooling green hue symbolizes renewal, grounding, and self-trust.

Mini Habit Challenge

Begin your morning without checking your phone.
Step outside, breathe deeply, and drink your Morning Glow Starter slowly.
Notice the light – and how refreshed your body feels from the inside out.

Affirmation of the Day

"I begin my day fresh, clear, and full of light.
Every sip renews my energy and my confidence."

Daily Notes Space:

01

How did you feel after today's morning smoothie? Any changes in energy, mood, or digestion?

DAY 2 – Green Goddess Reboot

Breakfast : Anti-Inflammatory Boost

- 1 cup kale leaves (stems removed)
- ½ green apple (cored)
- ½ cup fresh pineapple chunks
- ½ inch piece of fresh ginger (peeled)
- ½ lemon (peeled)
- 1 cup cold water or unsweetened coconut water
- Ice cubes (optional)

- Calories: ~110
- Natural Sugar: ~12g
- Key Nutrients:
- Vitamin C (pineapple, lemon) – supports collagen and immune defense
- Vitamin A & K (kale) – nourish skin and assist in detoxification
- Antioxidants (ginger) – reduce inflammation and support digestion
- Manganese (pineapple) – aids metabolism and energy production
- Fiber: ~4g

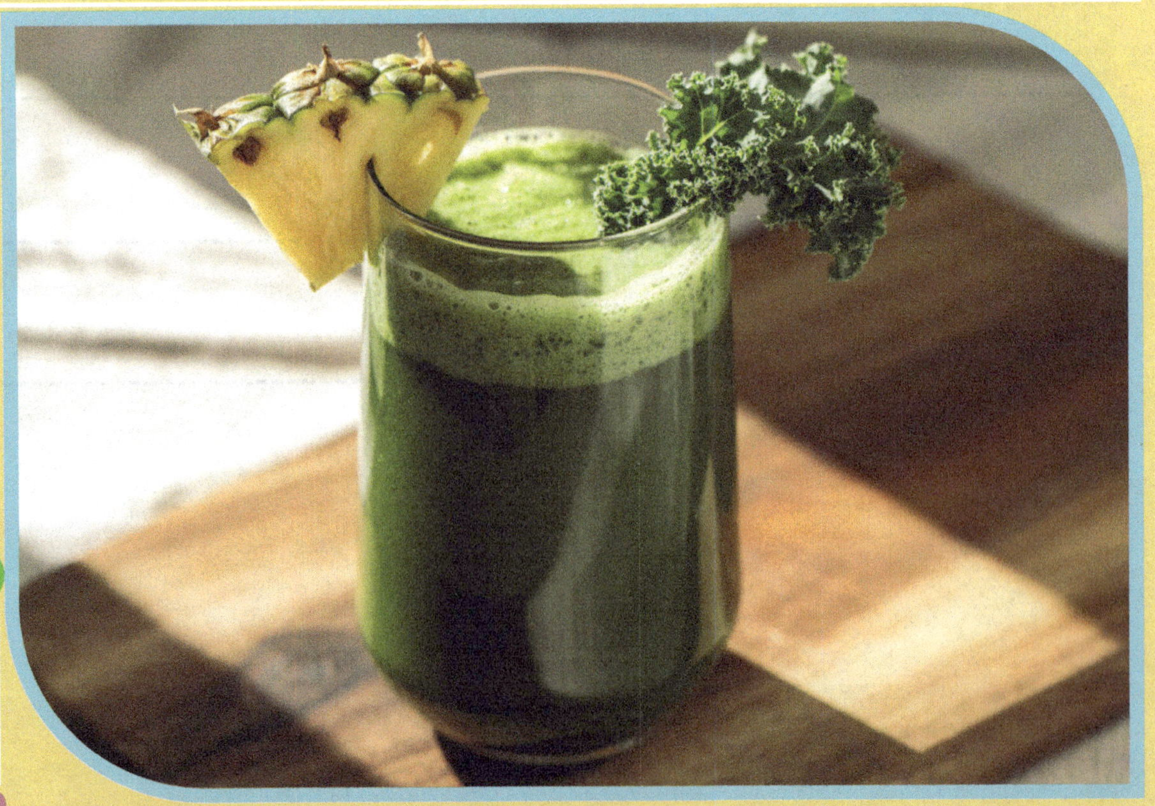

Find this recipe on our website

scan me

Nutritional & Health Benefits of Green Goddess Reboot

A Cleansing Boost for Digestion and Vitality

Your Green Goddess Reboot is your second step toward total renewal – a vibrant, earthy, and refreshing smoothie that reboots digestion and replenishes your cells with alkalizing minerals.

This blend helps your body continue releasing toxins while providing just the right balance of energy, hydration, and immune support.

By Day 2, your body is adjusting beautifully. You may feel lighter, clearer, and more awake – signs that your internal "reset" is already in motion.

Ingredient Power Breakdown

Kale – A nutritional powerhouse rich in chlorophyll, vitamin K, and fiber to cleanse and oxygenate the blood.

Green Apple – Adds a crisp sweetness while supporting gut health with natural pectin fiber.

Pineapple – Delivers bromelain enzymes for smooth digestion and glowing skin.

Lemon – Gently detoxifies the liver and boosts vitamin C for collagen production.

Ginger – Eases inflammation, reduces bloating, and stimulates circulation.

Coconut Water (Optional) – Adds electrolytes for hydration and post-detox balance.

Why It Matters for Women Over 40

The Green Goddess Reboot helps regulate digestion and hormone metabolism through fiber, minerals, and antioxidants.

It supports:

Hormonal detox by promoting liver and gut health

Reduced water retention and puffiness

Improved energy and clarity through natural electrolytes

Enhanced skin tone from vitamin C and chlorophyll synergy

This smoothie embodies the balance between power and grace – the essence of your day-two awakening.

Pro Tip:

Add a pinch of cayenne or extra ginger for a mild thermogenic effect that boosts metabolism and circulation naturally.

🌸 Mind-Body Connection & Lifestyle Insights

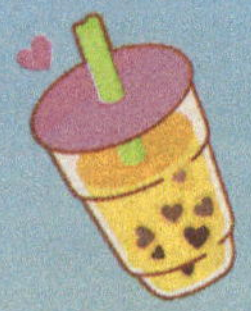

🌬 Today's Focus: Rejuvenation

Your body is remembering how to feel light again.

As you sip this bright-green blend, imagine every cell being rinsed clean and re-energized.

This isn't deprivation – it's liberation from heaviness, stress, and fatigue.

🧘 Mind-Body Benefits

Greens calm inflammation in both body and mood.

Ginger and lemon awaken digestion while sharpening mental clarity.

Mindful hydration strengthens your connection to calm awareness.

🌿 Mini Habit Challenge

After drinking your smoothie, take a brief walk outside.

Deep breathing in fresh air amplifies oxygen flow – extending your detox from your body to your mind.

💎 Affirmation of the Day

"I release what no longer serves me.

My body feels lighter, my mind feels clearer, and I am ready to shine."

Daily Notes Space:

02

Notice any difference in your digestion today? How did this smoothie make your body feel after breakfast or as a mid-morning drink?

DAY 3 – Tropical Detox Splash

Breakfast : Energy Lift & Tropical Cleanse

- 1 cup coconut water (unsweetened)
- ½ cup frozen mango chunks
- ½ small banana
- Juice of ½ lime
- 1 tablespoon chia seeds (optional, for fiber)
- 4–5 fresh mint leaves
- Ice cubes (as desired)

- Calories: ~150
- Natural Sugar: ~16g
- Key Nutrients:
- Vitamin C (mango, lime) – supports skin glow and immune function
- Potassium (banana, coconut water) – restores electrolyte balance
- Antioxidants (mint, mango) – fight free radicals and inflammation
- Fiber (chia seeds) – supports digestive regularity and satiety
- Fiber: ~5g

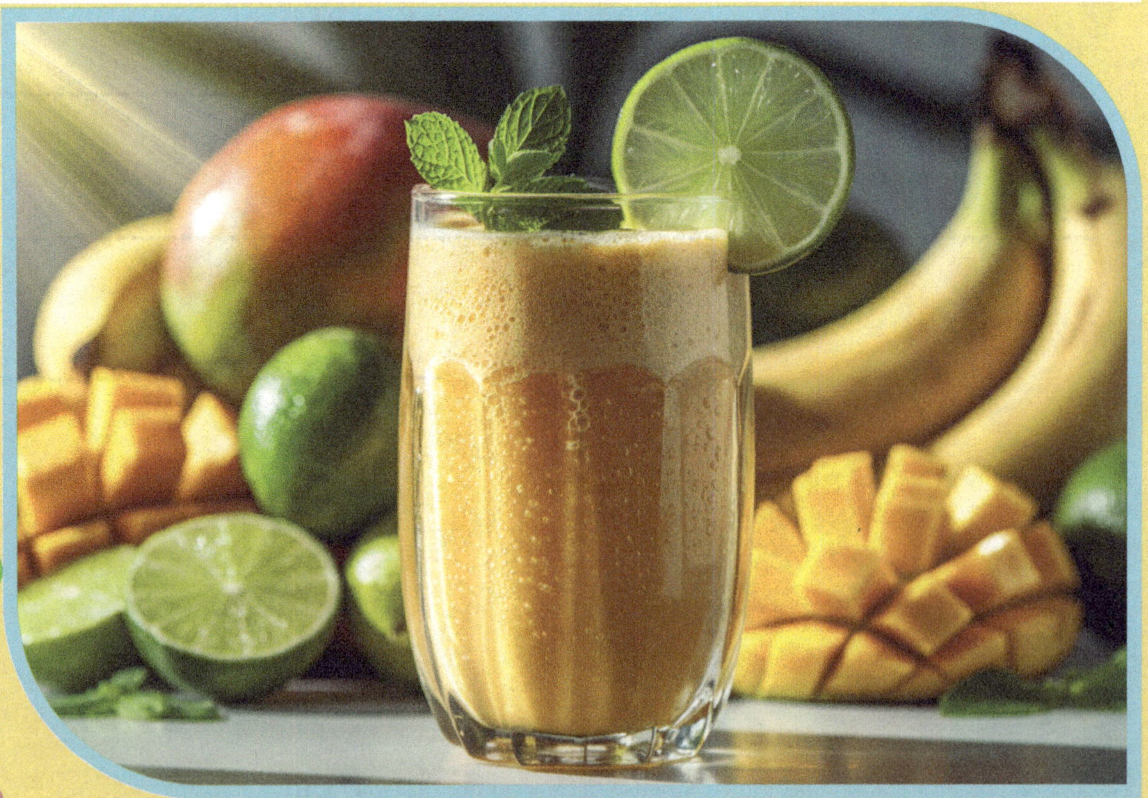

Find this recipe on our website

scan me

🌴 Nutritional & Health Benefits of Tropical Detox Splash

A Tropical Infusion for Lightness and Energy

Your Tropical Detox Splash Smoothie is like a mini island escape – hydrating, refreshing, and perfectly balanced to keep your body feeling light and your mind clear.

This tropical blend combines hydration, antioxidants, and digestive fiber to gently flush toxins while fueling natural energy.

By Day 3, your system is cleaner, your cravings are fading, and your body is embracing nourishment over excess. This smoothie keeps that momentum flowing – calm, bright, and deliciously simple.

Ingredient Power Breakdown

Coconut Water – Replenishes electrolytes, reduces fatigue, and supports kidney detox.
Mango – Delivers vitamin C and beta-carotene for glowing skin and immune health.
Banana – Adds potassium and smooth texture while stabilizing blood sugar.
Lime – Alkalizes the body and enhances collagen formation.
Chia Seeds (Optional) – Offer omega-3s and fiber for gentle digestive support.
Mint – Refreshes the palate, eases digestion, and cools inflammation.

Why It Matters for Women Over 40

The Tropical Detox Splash helps your body release water retention and support adrenal recovery – two key aspects of midlife balance.

It helps by:

Restoring electrolytes to combat fatigue and hormonal bloating
Supporting liver detox through citrus and antioxidants
Boosting collagen and skin elasticity with vitamin C
Providing anti-inflammatory hydration that enhances energy and clarity

This blend reminds you that cleansing doesn't mean restriction – it means renewal.

✨ Pro Tip:

Drink this smoothie slowly through a straw. Savoring each sip helps your digestion and hydration work in sync – enhancing nutrient absorption.

Mind-Body Connection & Lifestyle Insights

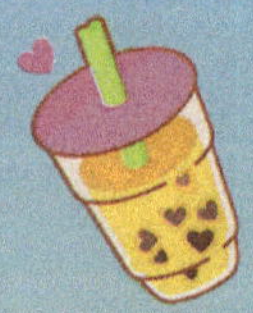

Today's Focus: Lightness & Joy

Your body is waking up, and so is your spirit.
As you sip this sunny, tropical blend, imagine letting go of yesterday's heaviness.
This smoothie is your morning reset – your first deep breath of the day, in liquid form.

Mind-Body Benefits

Combines hydration and antioxidants to lift mood and focus.
Invites mindfulness through cooling, tropical flavors.
Reminds your nervous system that nourishment can also feel joyful.

Mini Habit Challenge

Take five minutes in the morning to step outside into sunlight while drinking your smoothie.
Natural light tells your body to produce serotonin – your happiness hormone.

Affirmation of the Day

"I welcome lightness and joy into my day.
My energy flows freely, refreshed and renewed."

Daily Notes Space:

03

How did today's tropical blend make you feel? Did you notice better hydration or lighter digestion through the morning?

Page intentionally left blank

Thank you so much for reading this book!

We'd Love to hear from You

Review us on Amazon

★★★★★

Scan me

-OR-

Touch or Click here to review

DAY 4 – Citrus Cleanser

Lunch : Liver Cleanse & Immunity Boost

- 1 orange (peeled and seeded)
- ½ grapefruit (peeled and seeded)
- ½ cup fresh spinach leaves
- ½ frozen banana
- ½ cup unsweetened coconut water
- 1 teaspoon honey (optional, for taste)
- Ice cubes (optional)

- Calories: ~140
- Natural Sugar: ~14g
- Key Nutrients:
- Vitamin C (orange, grapefruit) – powerful immune booster and skin brightener
- Folate (spinach) – supports cellular repair and detox pathways
- Potassium (banana) – assists electrolyte balance and heart health
- Fiber (fruit pulp) – improves digestion and satiety
- Fiber: ~4g

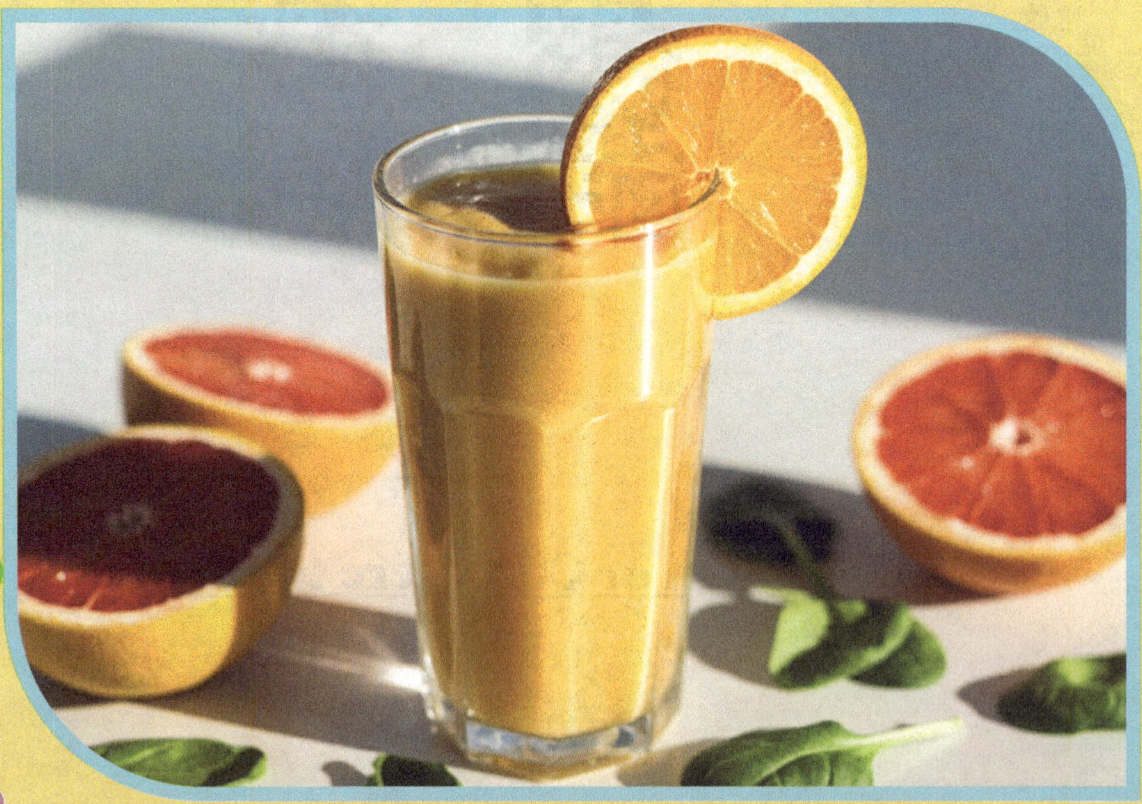

Find this recipe on our website

scan me

Nutritional & Health Benefits of Citrus Cleanser

A Zesty Reboot for Your Liver and Immunity

Your Citrus Cleanser Smoothie is a sunshine elixir – tart, tangy, and packed with cleansing power.

This radiant blend uses the detoxifying properties of citrus fruits to help your liver flush toxins while energizing your body with natural vitamin C and hydration.

By Day 4, your body is beginning to feel truly refreshed. The citrus enzymes are working behind the scenes to balance hormones, clear your skin, and fuel your vitality.

Ingredient Power Breakdown

Orange – Bursting with vitamin C to boost collagen, strengthen immunity, and promote youthful skin.

Grapefruit – Supports liver detoxification and fat metabolism while balancing blood sugar.

Spinach – Adds chlorophyll, folate, and iron to oxygenate your blood and enhance clarity.

Banana – Smooths texture and replenishes potassium for electrolyte balance.

Honey (Optional) – A touch of natural sweetness that soothes acidity and stabilizes energy.

Coconut Water (Optional) – Keeps your body hydrated and flushes out excess sodium.

Why It Matters for Women Over 40

Cleansing the liver and digestive system helps maintain hormone balance, especially during midlife transitions.

The Citrus Cleanser supports your system by:

Enhancing liver detox and fat metabolism

Boosting immune resilience through antioxidants

Supporting radiant, even-toned skin with vitamin C and hydration

Promoting a feeling of lightness and energy throughout the afternoon

This smoothie is your daily wake-up call – energizing, cleansing, and deeply restorative.

✨ Pro Tip:

Drink this smoothie midday, at least one hour before or after a heavy meal, to maximize nutrient absorption and liver efficiency.

Mind-Body Connection & Lifestyle Insights

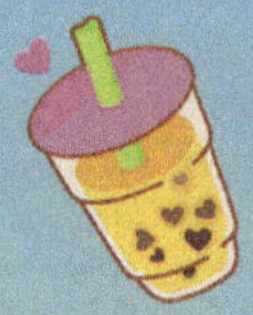

Today's Focus: Renewal

Your body is learning what balance feels like again – light, hydrated, and vibrant.
As you sip your citrus blend, imagine each drop clearing away yesterday's fatigue.
You are glowing from the inside out.

Mind-Body Benefits

The scent and color of citrus lift mood and relieve mental fog.
High vitamin C supports adrenal health, improving resilience to stress.
Gentle acids in citrus promote clarity – physically, mentally, and emotionally.

Mini Habit Challenge

Before drinking, close your eyes and inhale the citrus aroma deeply.
Let it awaken your senses and anchor your focus in the present moment.

Affirmation of the Day

"I am renewed, energized, and radiant.
Each sip fills me with clarity, balance, and joy."

Daily Notes Space:

04

Did this citrus combo give you an energy lift? Note how your skin and digestion feel by evening.

DAY 5 – Sweet Green Calm

Early Dinner (before 6 p.m.) : Evening Reset

- 1 cup fresh spinach leaves
- ½ ripe avocado
- 1 small banana
- 1 tablespoon chia seeds
- 1 cup unsweetened almond milk (or oat milk)
- ½ teaspoon pure vanilla extract (optional)
- Ice cubes (as desired)

- Calories: ~230
- Natural Sugar: ~10 g
- Key Nutrients:
  - Healthy monounsaturated fats (avocado) – support heart and hormonal health
  - Magnesium (spinach, chia) – relaxes muscles and reduces stress tension
  - Potassium (banana) – balances fluids and reduces evening bloat
  - Omega-3s (chia seeds) – anti-inflammatory and brain-nourishing
- Fiber: ~7 g

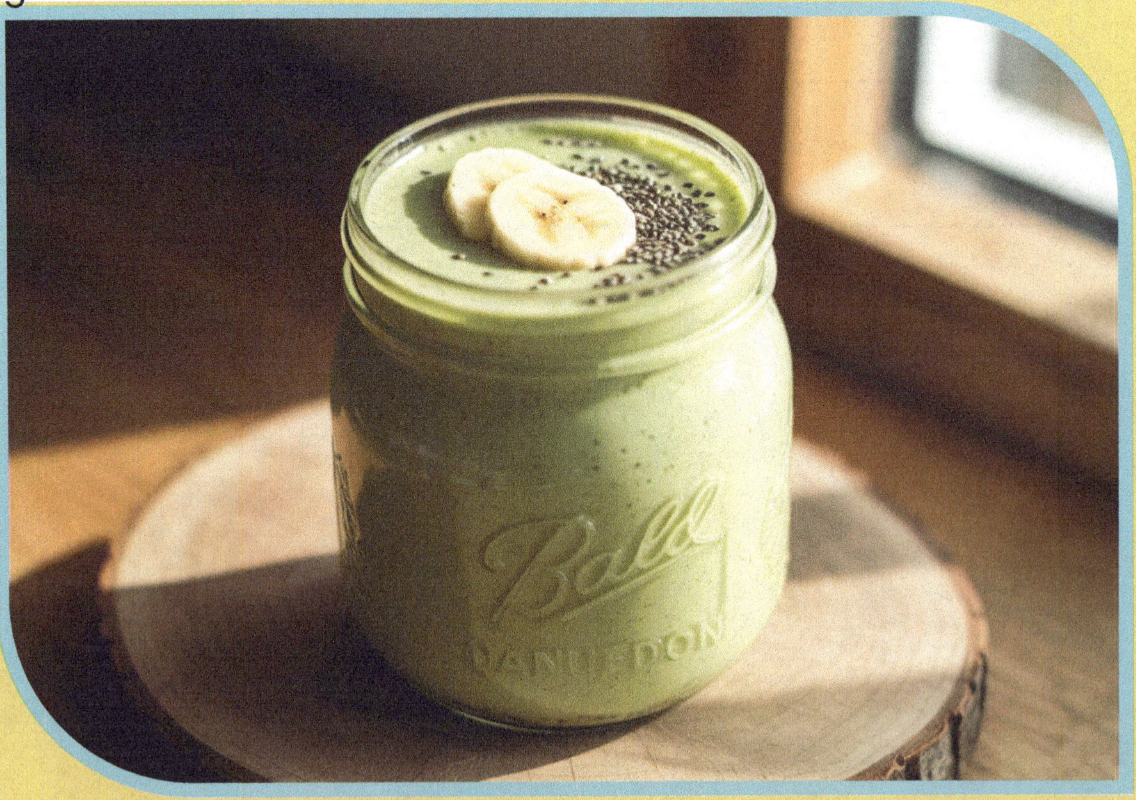

Find this recipe on our website

scan me

Nutritional & Health Benefits of Sweet Green Calm

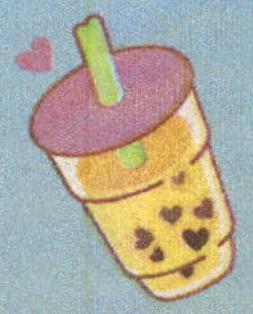

A Silky Blend for Calm, Balance, and Evening Renewal

Your Sweet Green Calm Smoothie is the definition of peaceful nourishment – creamy, soothing, and deeply satisfying.

This evening blend focuses on magnesium, omega-3s, and healthy fats that restore your nervous system, promote hormone balance, and prepare your body for deep, restful recovery overnight.

By Day 5, your detox rhythm is established – your energy is steady, your digestion smoother, and your sleep quality improving. This smoothie helps lock in that calm equilibrium.

Ingredient Power Breakdown

Spinach – High in magnesium and folate to support relaxation and cellular repair.

Avocado – Provides monounsaturated fats for heart and hormone health, plus vitamin E for radiant skin.

Banana – Adds potassium to release fluid retention and relax muscles.

Chia Seeds – Offer omega-3s and fiber to soothe inflammation and stabilize mood.

Almond or Oat Milk – Adds calcium and vitamin D for bone and muscle recovery.

Vanilla (Optional) – Enhances the creamy flavor while calming the senses.

Why It Matters for Women Over 40

This smoothie is designed to counteract the effects of stress and hormonal fluctuations that can disrupt digestion, sleep, and mood.

It helps by:

Easing stress-induced inflammation and muscle tension

Supporting stable blood sugar for evening calm

Promoting hormone balance through healthy fats and magnesium

Encouraging overnight repair and restful sleep

This is your evening exhale – smooth, satisfying, and restorative.

Pro Tip:

Drink this smoothie 1–2 hours before bed. The magnesium, potassium, and healthy fats work synergistically to relax your nervous system and help you wake up refreshed.

🌙 Mind-Body Connection & Lifestyle Insights

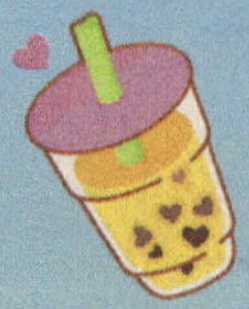

🌊 Today's Focus: Calm & Recovery

Your body is not asking for less – it's asking for balance.
As you sip this silky green smoothie, picture tension melting away.
You're not just nourishing your body; you're retraining your nervous system to choose calm over chaos.

🧘‍♀️ Mind-Body Benefits

Magnesium and omega-3s ease stress and anxiety.
Smooth, creamy texture encourages slow, mindful sipping.
Calming flavors of avocado and vanilla soothe emotional restlessness.

🧚 Mini Habit Challenge

End your evening screen-free for at least 30 minutes after your smoothie.
Let stillness – not stimulation – guide your body into recovery mode.

🖤 Affirmation of the Day

"I end my day nourished and peaceful.
Every choice I make brings me closer to balance."

Daily Notes Space:

05

Did this evening smoothie help you wind down? Note any changes in sleep quality or next-morning energy.

DAY 6 – Beet the Bloat

Breakfast : Circulation Boost

- ½ medium beetroot (peeled and chopped)
- 1 small apple (cored)
- 1 small carrot (peeled and chopped)
- Juice of ½ lemon
- ½ inch piece fresh ginger (peeled)
- ¾ cup cold water or coconut water
- Ice cubes (optional)

- Calories: ~130
- Natural Sugar: ~13 g
- Key Nutrients:
- Nitrates (beetroot) – support blood flow and natural energy
- Beta-carotene (carrot) – promotes skin health and vision
- Vitamin C (lemon, apple) – supports collagen and immune repair
- Fiber (apple, beet) – aids digestion and natural detox pathways
- Fiber: ~4 g

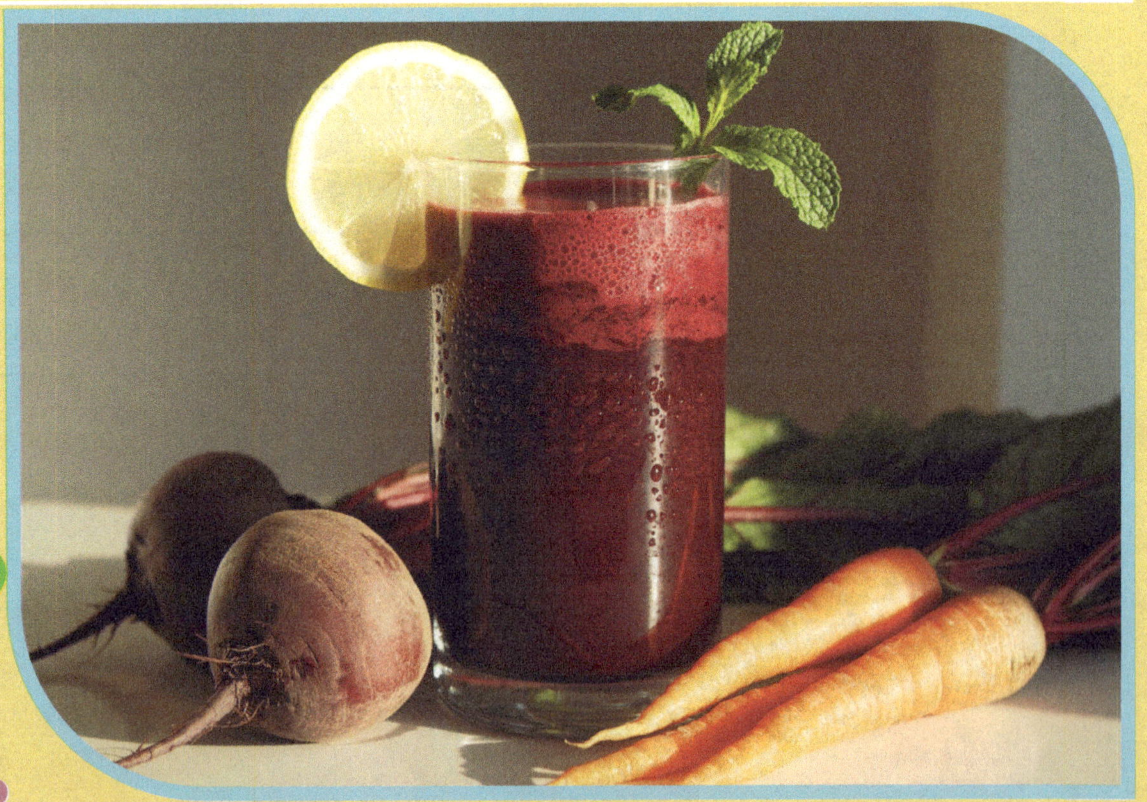

Find this recipe on our website

scan me

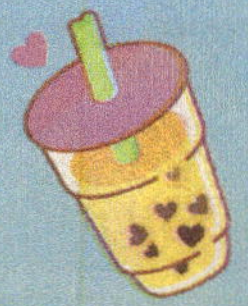

Nutritional & Health Benefits of Beet the Bloat

A Vibrant Detox for Energy and Circulation

Your Beet the Bloat Smoothie is as beautiful as it is powerful – a vivid, magenta-colored elixir that energizes your body, flushes excess water, and promotes deep cellular renewal.

This blend stimulates blood flow, enhances oxygen delivery, and clears out toxins that often leave you feeling puffy or fatigued.

By Day 6, your detox systems – liver, lymph, and gut – are all in motion. This smoothie helps them function smoothly, giving you the kind of glow that starts from within.

Ingredient Power Breakdown

Beetroot – Rich in nitrates that expand blood vessels and boost stamina while aiding liver detox.

Apple – Adds gentle sweetness and soluble fiber to regulate digestion.

Carrot – Offers beta-carotene for glowing skin and eye health.

Lemon – Provides vitamin C to brighten complexion and support collagen synthesis.

Ginger – Reduces inflammation, stimulates circulation, and aids digestion.

Coconut Water (Optional) – Restores electrolytes and assists detox hydration.

Why It Matters for Women Over 40

This rejuvenating blend helps reset circulation, energy, and digestion – three key systems that slow with age.

It supports:

Hormonal balance through improved blood oxygenation

Liver detox and natural bloat reduction

Healthier skin tone through enhanced nutrient delivery

Mid-morning energy without caffeine or sugar spikes

This smoothie proves that clean living can be colorful, satisfying, and revitalizing.

Pro Tip:

Drink your beet smoothie slowly and cold. The nitrates activate best when sipped gradually, allowing your body to fully absorb their circulation-enhancing benefits.

Mind-Body Connection & Lifestyle Insights

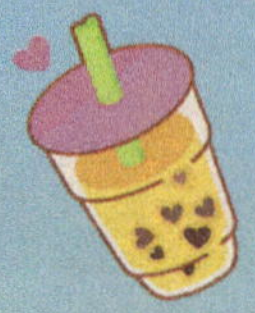

Today's Focus: Circulation & Flow

Your energy isn't just inside you – it flows through you.

As you sip this bold, magenta smoothie, imagine your body's channels opening – fresh oxygen, light, and vitality reaching every cell.

This is nourishment that moves.

Mind-Body Benefits

Improves mental clarity through better blood and oxygen flow.

Beetroot's color and compounds energize the heart chakra – your center of love and connection.

Encourages mindfulness through visual beauty and rich, earthy flavor.

Mini Habit Challenge

Before your first sip, take three deep breaths and stretch your arms wide – opening your chest and shoulders.

Better posture means better oxygen flow and stronger energy all day.

Affirmation of the Day

"I am open, flowing, and energized.

My body is light, my heart is strong, and my energy moves with ease."

Daily Notes Space:

06

Did you notice lighter digestion or improved morning energy? Write how this bright blend made you feel.

DAY 7 – Hydration Healer

Lunch : Deep Hydration & Skin Radiance

- 1½ cups watermelon cubes (seedless)
- Juice of ½ lime
- 5–6 fresh mint leaves
- ½ cup cucumber slices
- ½ cup cold coconut water
- Ice cubes (optional)

- Calories: ~90
- Natural Sugar: ~10 g
- Key Nutrients:
- Lycopene (watermelon) – antioxidant that supports heart and skin health
- Vitamin C (lime) – strengthens immune defense and boosts collagen
- Potassium (coconut water) – maintains fluid balance
- Hydration compounds (cucumber, watermelon) – replenish electrolytes naturally
- Fiber: ~2 g

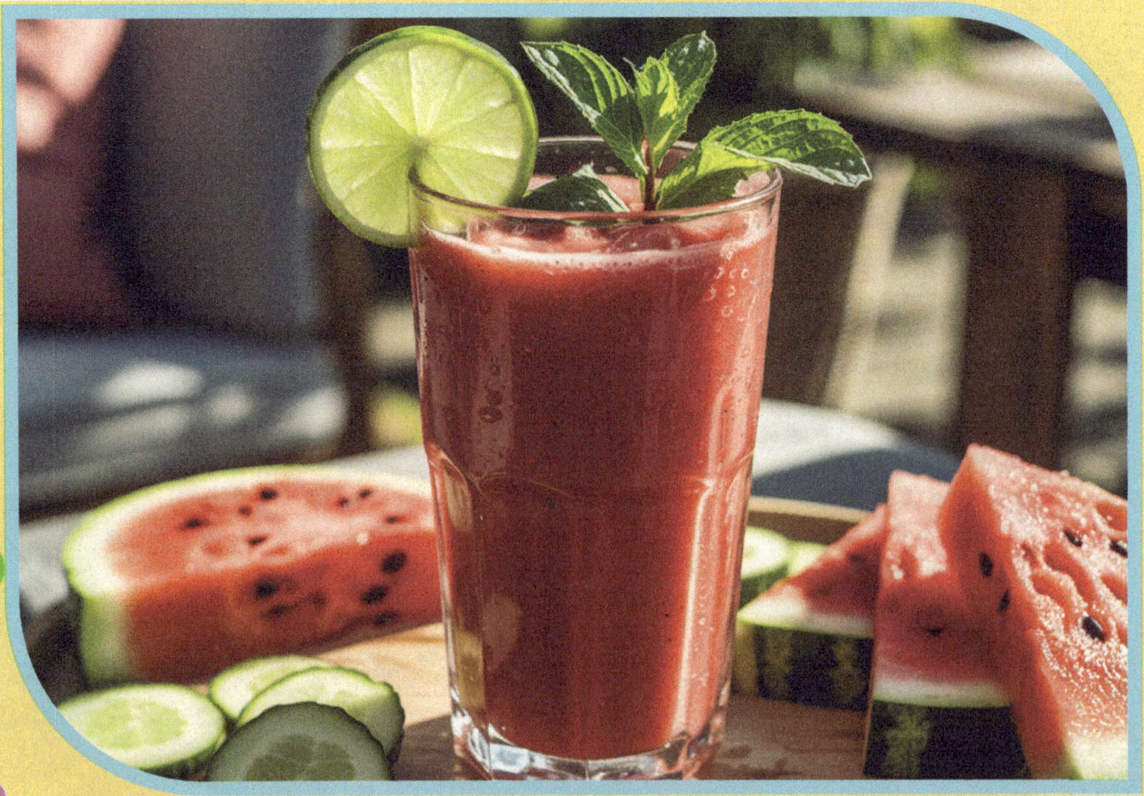

Find this recipe on our website

scan me

💧 Nutritional & Health Benefits of Hydration Healer

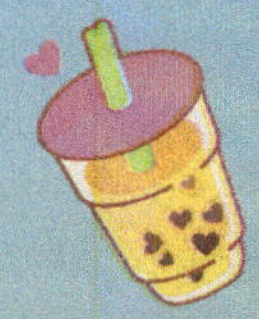

✂ A Cooling Elixir for Deep Hydration and Radiance

Your Hydration Healer Smoothie is your body's gentle reset button – crisp, juicy, and perfectly balanced to restore electrolytes, soothe inflammation, and keep your skin glowing. This blend is naturally low in calories but high in essential hydration compounds that replenish cells, aid detox, and promote elasticity in the skin.

By Day 7, your system is clearer, lighter, and more balanced. The week's cleansing phase completes with this refreshing elixir – a true hydration celebration from the inside out.

Ingredient Power Breakdown

Watermelon – Packed with lycopene and hydration compounds that support heart health and radiant skin.

Cucumber – High in silica and water content to cool inflammation and rehydrate tissues.

Lime – Adds vitamin C for collagen production and gentle detoxification.

Mint – Refreshes digestion and invigorates the senses.

Coconut Water – Delivers natural electrolytes to rebalance energy and reduce fatigue.

✿ Why It Matters for Women Over 40

Hydration becomes harder to maintain with age due to hormonal shifts and slower cellular renewal. This smoothie helps:

Reduce puffiness and water retention naturally

Enhance skin moisture and elasticity through hydration and vitamin C

Improve focus and energy by replenishing lost electrolytes

Calm inflammation and support smoother digestion

The Hydration Healer proves that beauty truly begins with balance and water – nature's purest detox.

✨ Pro Tip:

Drink this smoothie mid-day or after light activity. The blend of potassium, vitamin C, and water-rich fruits helps your body recover faster and maintain consistent hydration.

Mind-Body Connection & Lifestyle Insights

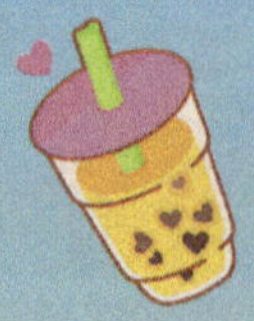

Today's Focus: Refresh & Reconnect

Your body speaks through sensation – thirst, tightness, fatigue.
This smoothie teaches you to listen and respond with compassion.
As you sip, imagine every cell lighting up, every organ sighing with relief.

Mind-Body Benefits

Rehydrates at the cellular level, reducing fatigue and mental fog.
The cooling combination of mint and cucumber soothes the nervous system.
The light sweetness of watermelon promotes emotional balance and calm joy.

Mini Habit Challenge

Before blending, fill a glass with water and drink it mindfully.
Feel how your body thanks you for each sip – and let hydration become your daily ritual of care.

Affirmation of the Day

"I am refreshed, radiant, and deeply hydrated.
My body glows with energy, and my spirit flows with ease."

Daily Notes Space:

07

How hydrated did you feel after this lunch replacement? Note any changes in skin glow or afternoon energy levels.

DAY 8 – Berry Power Fuel

Breakfast for Antioxidant Defense

- ½ cup frozen blueberries
- ½ cup frozen strawberries
- 1 small banana
- 2 tablespoons rolled oats
- 1 cup unsweetened almond milk (or oat milk)
- 1 teaspoon honey or agave (optional)
- Ice cubes (optional)

- Calories: ~210
- Natural Sugar: ~15 g
- Key Nutrients:
- Antioxidants (blueberries, strawberries) – protect cells and support skin health
- Potassium (banana) – restores electrolytes after morning fasting
- Fiber & beta-glucans (oats) – improve digestion and regulate blood sugar
- Calcium & Vitamin E (almond milk) – support bone and skin health
- Fiber: ~6 g

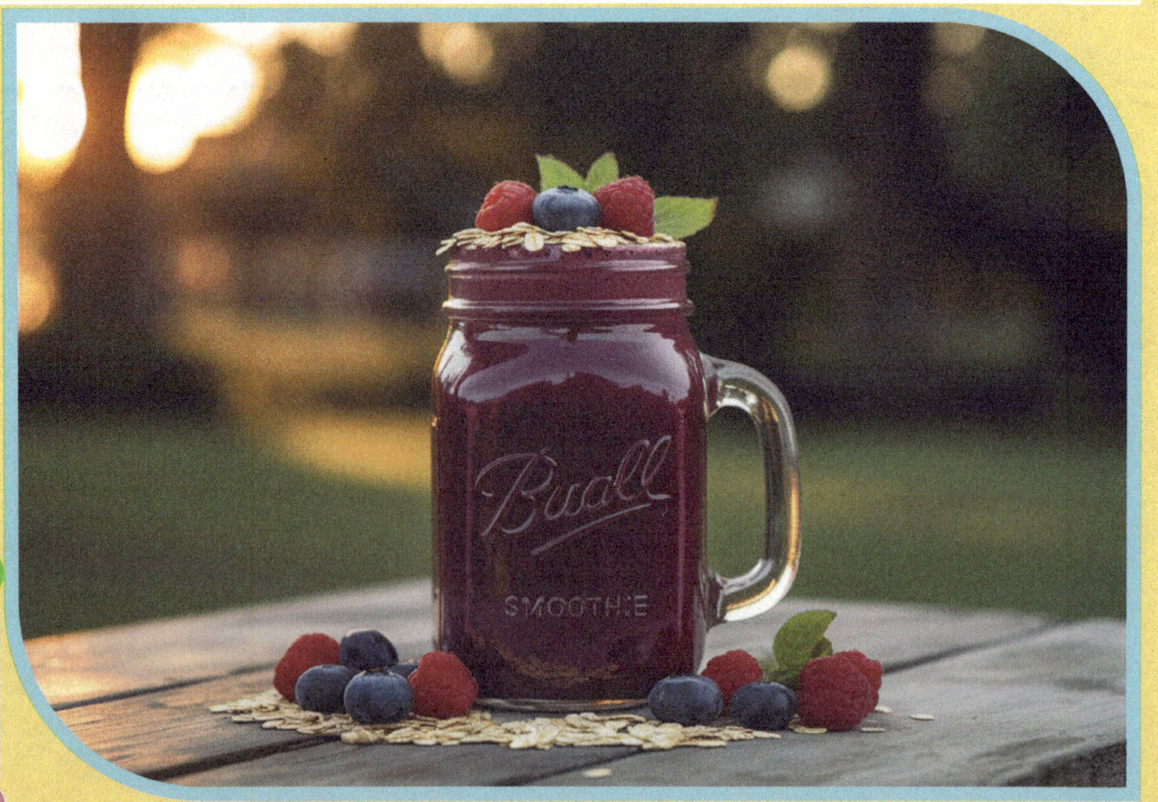

Find this recipe on our website

scan me

Nutritional & Health Benefits of Berry Power Fuel

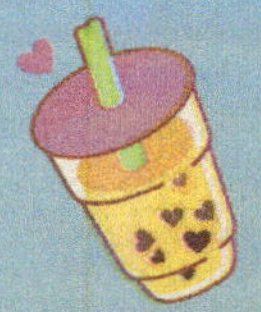

A Morning Boost to Energize and Rebuild

Your Berry Power Fuel smoothie is a morning favorite – rich, creamy, and deeply satisfying. It's designed to rebuild your energy reserves after a night of fasting while flooding your body with antioxidants that protect, repair, and renew.

By Day 8, your metabolism has awakened; this blend helps maintain momentum so you feel strong, sharp, and balanced all day.

Ingredient Power Breakdown

Blueberries – High in anthocyanins that fight free-radical damage and support memory, heart, and skin health.

Strawberries – Packed with vitamin C for collagen production and brighter skin tone.

Banana – Provides potassium to restore electrolytes and steady morning energy.

Rolled Oats – Add soluble fiber that stabilizes blood sugar and keeps you full for hours.

Unsweetened Almond Milk – Light, low-calorie calcium source; vitamin E protects skin and hormones.

Honey or Agave (Optional) – A gentle, natural sweetener that enhances taste without spikes.

Why It Matters for Women Over 40

As estrogen shifts, energy and glucose balance can fluctuate. This smoothie helps by:

Providing slow-release carbohydrates for sustained focus

Supporting collagen, bone, and skin health with antioxidants and calcium

Promoting digestive balance through beta-glucans and fiber

Rebuilding morning energy without caffeine

This is your steady-energy formula – the perfect way to start the day nourished, not rushed.

Pro Tip:

For extra staying power, sprinkle chia or flax on top for added omega-3s and texture.

Mind-Body Connection & Lifestyle Insights

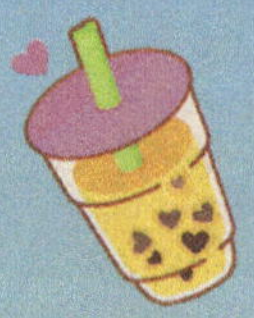

Today's Focus: Energize & Rebuild

Your body is learning to trust you again – you feed it, it fuels you back.

As you enjoy this deep-purple smoothie, think of energy not as speed, but as stability.

You're building stamina, patience, and self-respect one choice at a time.

Mind-Body Benefits

Nutrient-dense carbs + fiber = consistent focus and fewer mood dips.

Deep berry pigments nurture brain vitality and intuition.

The mindful act of breakfasting with purpose rewires your morning rhythm toward calm energy.

Mini Habit Challenge

Before you check your phone, take three slow breaths and drink the first half of your smoothie in silence.

Let stillness, not stress, set your tone for the day.

Affirmation of the Day

"I begin my day balanced, nourished, and strong.

My energy flows smoothly and supports everything I choose to do."

Daily Notes Space:

08

Did this smoothie keep you full until lunchtime? Note your energy and focus levels this morning.

DAY 9 – Sunshine Glow

Lunch : Inflammation Relief & Skin Radiance

- 1 cup frozen mango chunks
- ½ banana
- ½ teaspoon ground turmeric (or ½ inch fresh turmeric root, peeled)
- ½ inch piece of fresh ginger (peeled)
- 1 teaspoon honey (optional)
- 1 cup unsweetened almond milk (or coconut milk)
- Ice cubes (optional)

- Calories: ~180
- Natural Sugar: ~14 g
- Key Nutrients:
- Curcumin (turmeric) – powerful anti-inflammatory and antioxidant
- Vitamin A & C (mango) – promote skin glow and immune health
- Potassium (banana) – maintains hydration and muscle balance
- Gingerol (ginger) – supports digestion and reduces bloating
- Fiber: ~4 g

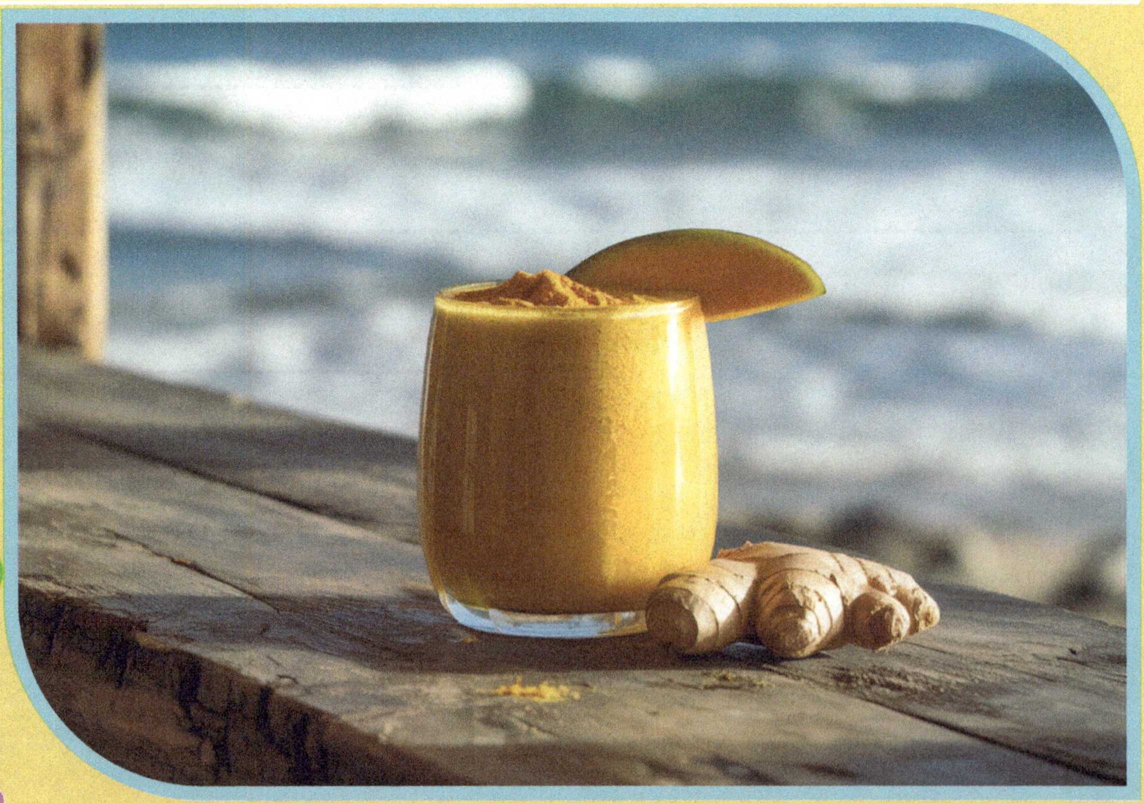

Find this recipe on our website

scan me

Nutritional & Health Benefits of Sunshine Glow

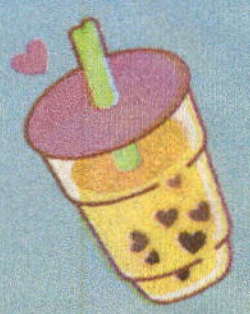

A Radiant Reset from the Inside Out

Your Sunshine Glow Smoothie is like a golden sunrise in a glass – creamy, bright, and full of rejuvenating nutrients.

This tropical blend helps fight inflammation, balance hydration, and awaken your skin's natural radiance. By Day 9, your body is no longer in "detox mode" – it's in rebuild mode, restoring strength and glow with every sip.

Ingredient Power Breakdown

Mango – Rich in vitamin A, beta-carotene, and vitamin C for vibrant, healthy skin and immune support.

Banana – Provides potassium to maintain electrolyte balance and prevent muscle fatigue.

Turmeric – Contains curcumin, a natural anti-inflammatory compound that promotes joint comfort and skin clarity.

Ginger – Aids digestion, reduces bloating, and boosts circulation for that natural post-detox glow.

Honey (Optional) – Adds mild sweetness and antibacterial benefits.

Almond or Coconut Milk – Hydrating, calcium-rich base with a creamy tropical texture.

Why It Matters for Women Over 40

The combination of antioxidants, electrolytes, and anti-inflammatory compounds in this smoothie helps:

Ease joint stiffness and hormonal inflammation

Support glowing, firm skin through vitamin A and C synergy

Improve gut health for clearer, more radiant complexion

Rebuild natural energy and muscle tone post-detox

This blend reminds your body what balance feels like – strong, fluid, and bright.

Pro Tip:

Blend turmeric with a pinch of black pepper – it boosts curcumin absorption up to 2000%.

🌼 Mind-Body Connection & Lifestyle Insights

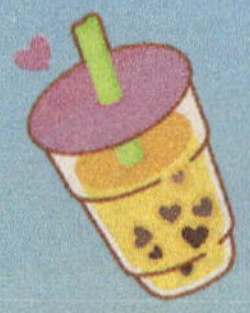

🌤 Today's Focus: Radiance

You've nourished, cleansed, and balanced – now it's time to shine.

As you sip your golden smoothie, think of your body as sunlight in motion. Every cell is absorbing warmth, light, and renewal.

You're not chasing glow – you're becoming it.

🧘 Mind-Body Benefits

Bright color therapy (yellow-gold) uplifts mood and boosts confidence.

Anti-inflammatory ingredients calm both physical and emotional tension.

The simple act of savoring something beautiful reconnects you to gratitude.

✨ Mini Habit Challenge

Write down three moments that made you smile today – no matter how small.

Joy is the most potent beauty serum there is.

💎 Affirmation of the Day

"I radiate warmth, strength, and beauty from within.

My glow is the reflection of balance and joy."

Daily Notes Space:

09

Did you notice a lift in mood or energy today? Note any changes in digestion or skin brightness after this smoothie.

Page intentionally left blank

Thank you so much for reading this book!

We'd Love to hear from You

Review us on Amazon

Scan me

-OR-

Touch or Click here to review

DAY 10 – Skin Saver Smoothie

Early Dinner (before 6 p.m.) : Skin Renewal

- 1 cup fresh or frozen strawberries
- ½ cup plain Greek yogurt (unsweetened)
- 1 small banana
- 1 tablespoon collagen powder (unflavored or vanilla)
- 1 teaspoon flaxseed oil or ground flaxseed
- ¾ cup unsweetened almond milk (or milk of choice)
- Ice cubes (optional)

- Calories: ~210
- Natural Sugar: ~12 g
- Key Nutrients:
- Collagen peptides – support skin elasticity and reduce fine lines
- Vitamin C (strawberries, banana) – aids collagen absorption and brightens complexion
- Protein & probiotics (Greek yogurt) – strengthen gut-skin connection
- Omega-3s (flaxseed) – maintain moisture barrier and reduce inflammation
- Fiber: ~4 g

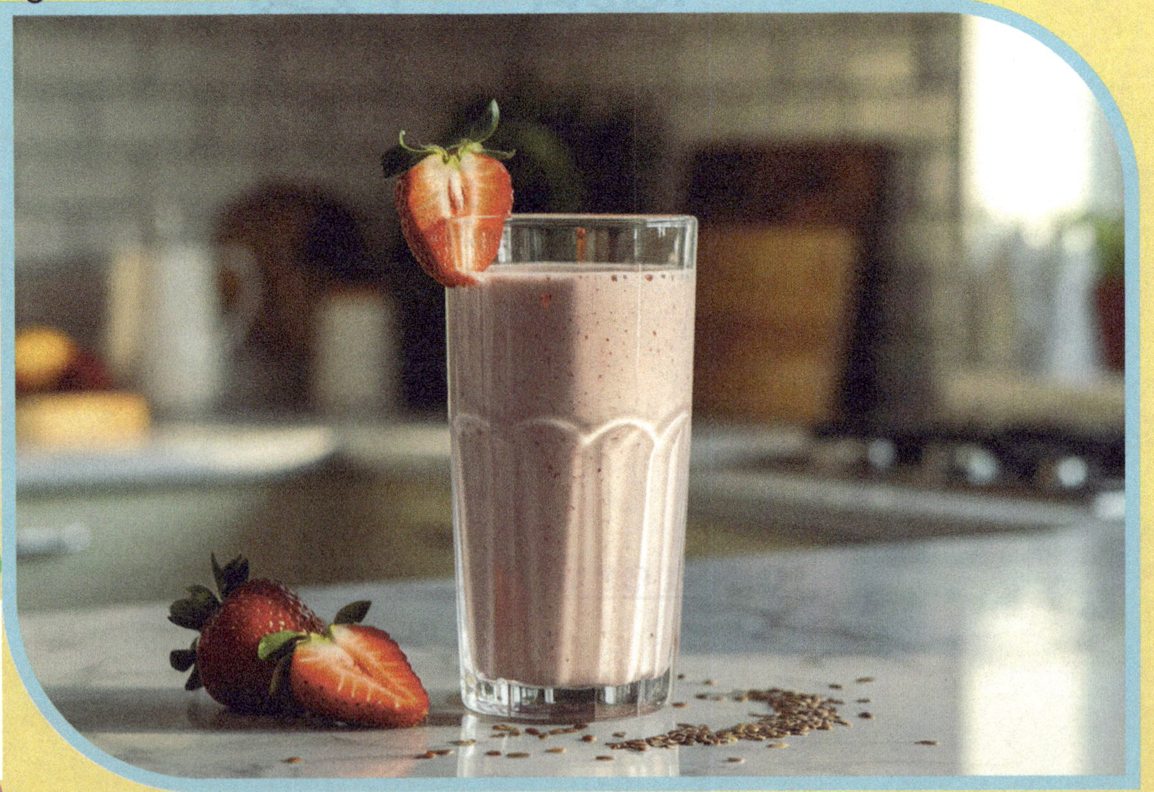

Find this recipe on our website

scan me

❤ Nutritional & Health Benefits of Skin Saver Smoothie

💕 A Creamy Blend for Beauty and Recovery

The Skin Saver Smoothie is your inside-out skincare ritual – rich, silky, and designed to restore elasticity, radiance, and calm.

By Day 10, your detox has balanced your system; now it's time to feed your skin what it truly needs: collagen, hydration, and anti-inflammatory fats that work while you rest.

This smoothie blends nutrients that support overnight repair, reduce fine lines, and replenish the glow your body has been building since Day 1.

Ingredient Power Breakdown

Strawberries – Loaded with vitamin C to aid collagen synthesis and brighten complexion.

Greek Yogurt – A source of protein and probiotics that fortify the gut-skin connection.

Banana – Adds potassium for hydration and natural smoothness to skin texture.

Collagen Powder – Supports elasticity, reduces fine lines, and strengthens hair and nails.

Flaxseed Oil (or Ground Flax) – Omega-3s help maintain skin's moisture barrier and calm inflammation.

Almond Milk – Provides vitamin E for antioxidant skin protection.

Why It Matters for Women Over 40

Collagen production naturally declines after 35, leading to dryness, fine lines, and uneven tone.

The Skin Saver Smoothie helps your body:

Rebuild collagen from within for firmer, more supple skin

Calm redness and puffiness through omega-3s

Improve digestion for clearer, more even complexion

Support hormonal balance that affects skin tone and hydration

This blend is your nightly beauty routine – in smoothie form.

✨ Pro Tip:

Drink this smoothie 2–3 hours before bedtime to give your body time to digest, absorb nutrients, and begin overnight repair while you sleep.

Mind-Body Connection & Lifestyle Insights

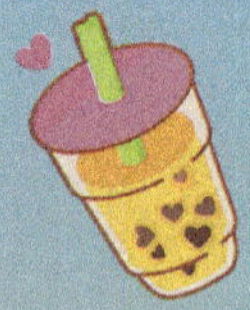

Today's Focus: Nourish & Restore

Your body repairs itself best when it's calm – so tonight, you nourish both peace and beauty. As you sip this soothing pink blend, picture your cells relaxing into renewal. Your skin isn't aging – it's responding to care.

Mind-Body Benefits

Encourages self-kindness through mindful evening rituals.
Combines nutrition and relaxation to lower cortisol – a key skin-aging trigger.
Supports emotional grounding through warm, nurturing flavors.

Mini Habit Challenge

After your smoothie, wash your face gently, hydrate your skin, and take five slow breaths in the mirror.
Affirm your worth – because self-care is beauty care.

Affirmation of the Day

"I treat my body and skin with love.
Radiance is the reflection of how gently I care for myself."

Daily Notes Space:

10

How did your skin feel after this smoothie? Any noticeable glow or hydration boost this morning? Record your thoughts here.

DAY 11 – Vanilla Protein Dream

Breakfast : Muscle Support & Metabolic Boost

- 1 scoop vanilla protein powder (plant-based or whey)
- 1 tablespoon almond butter
- 1 small banana
- 1 cup unsweetened almond milk (or milk of choice)
- ½ teaspoon cinnamon (optional)
- ½ teaspoon pure vanilla extract
- Ice cubes (optional)

- Calories: ~240
- Natural Sugar: ~8 g
- Key Nutrients:
- Protein (powder + almond butter) – supports muscle repair and boosts metabolism
- Magnesium (almonds) – promotes calm focus and energy balance
- Potassium (banana) – aids hydration and nerve function
- Healthy fats (almond butter) – improve satiety and hormone balance
- Fiber: ~4 g

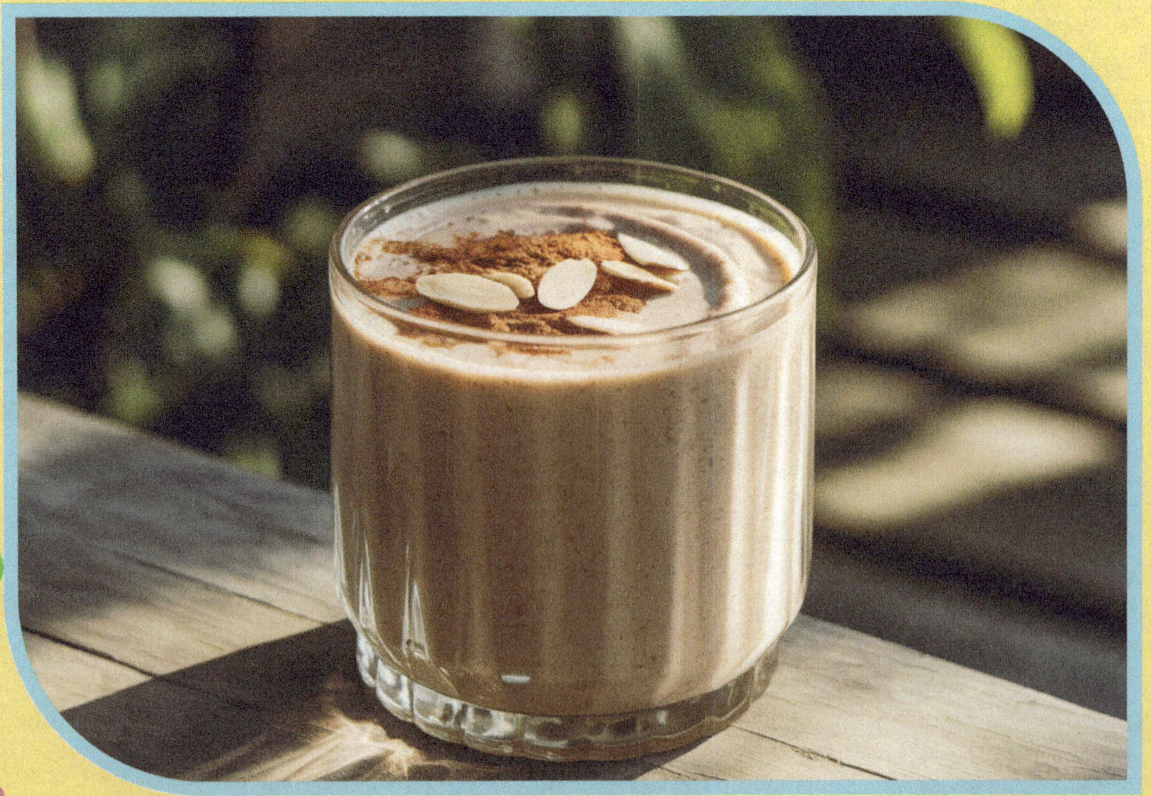

Find this recipe on our website

scan me

💪 Nutritional & Health Benefits of Vanilla Protein Dream

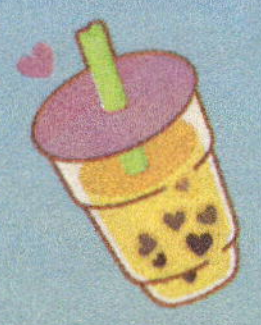

🖤 A Smooth Start for Strength and Focus

Your Vanilla Protein Dream is a creamy, balanced breakfast that builds muscle tone, stabilizes blood sugar, and sets a calm, confident tone for your day.

By Day 11, your metabolism is active and balanced — now it's time to fuel it.

This smoothie provides the perfect harmony of protein, healthy fats, and minerals to sustain you through your morning with steady, focused energy.

🍌 Ingredient Power Breakdown

Vanilla Protein Powder – Supplies complete amino acids for lean muscle repair and lasting fullness.

Almond Butter – Adds healthy fats and magnesium to improve mood, brain focus, and hormone balance.

Banana – Provides potassium to support hydration, nerve function, and muscle relaxation.

Almond Milk – Light and low in calories, offering calcium and vitamin E for skin and bone health.

Cinnamon (Optional) – Naturally balances blood sugar and supports circulation.

Vanilla Extract – Enhances flavor while offering mild antioxidant properties.

🌸 Why It Matters for Women Over 40

As we age, muscle tone and metabolism naturally slow — leading to energy dips and cravings.

The Vanilla Protein Dream helps your body:

Maintain lean muscle mass and metabolic efficiency

Support hormone production through healthy fats

Curb cravings and sustain fullness until lunch

Promote calm focus and reduced stress through magnesium and balanced blood sugar

This smoothie is your morning armor — light, creamy, and empowering.

✨ Pro Tip:

If using plant-based protein, add a few drops of pure vanilla extract or a pinch of sea salt to round out the flavor profile naturally.

Mind-Body Connection & Lifestyle Insights

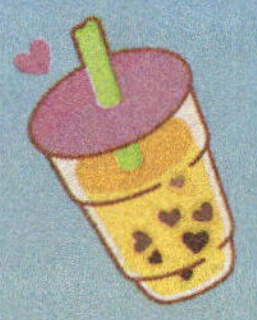

Today's Focus: Strength & Stability

This smoothie represents foundation – nourishment that's steady, simple, and strong. As you sip, think about the kind of energy you want to carry today – focused, grounded, and unshakeable.

Mind-Body Benefits

Protein helps balance cortisol, supporting emotional stability.
Magnesium promotes calm alertness – energy without anxiety.
Satisfying healthy fats signal safety and reduce emotional eating triggers.

Mini Habit Challenge

Before your first sip, stand tall and take three slow breaths.
Say aloud: "I'm choosing strength today."
This simple grounding moment transforms your breakfast into a mindset ritual.

Affirmation of the Day

"I am strong, balanced, and focused.
My energy supports me in every way I choose to move."

Daily Notes Space:

11

Did this smoothie keep your hunger steady until lunch? Track how your energy and mood felt through the morning.

DAY 12 – Carrot Cake Energizer

Lunch : Hormone Balance & Afternoon Energy

- 1 medium carrot (peeled and chopped)
- ½ frozen banana
- 2 tablespoons rolled oats
- ½ teaspoon cinnamon
- ½ teaspoon vanilla extract
- 1 cup unsweetened almond milk (or oat milk)
- 1 teaspoon honey or maple syrup (optional)
- Ice cubes (optional)

- Calories: ~190
- Natural Sugar: ~12 g
- Key Nutrients:
- Beta-carotene (carrots) – supports skin, eye, and immune health
- Fiber (oats, banana) – promotes digestive balance and fullness
- Cinnamon – helps regulate blood sugar and reduce cravings
- Vitamin B6 (banana) – assists metabolism and nervous system support
- Fiber: ~5 g

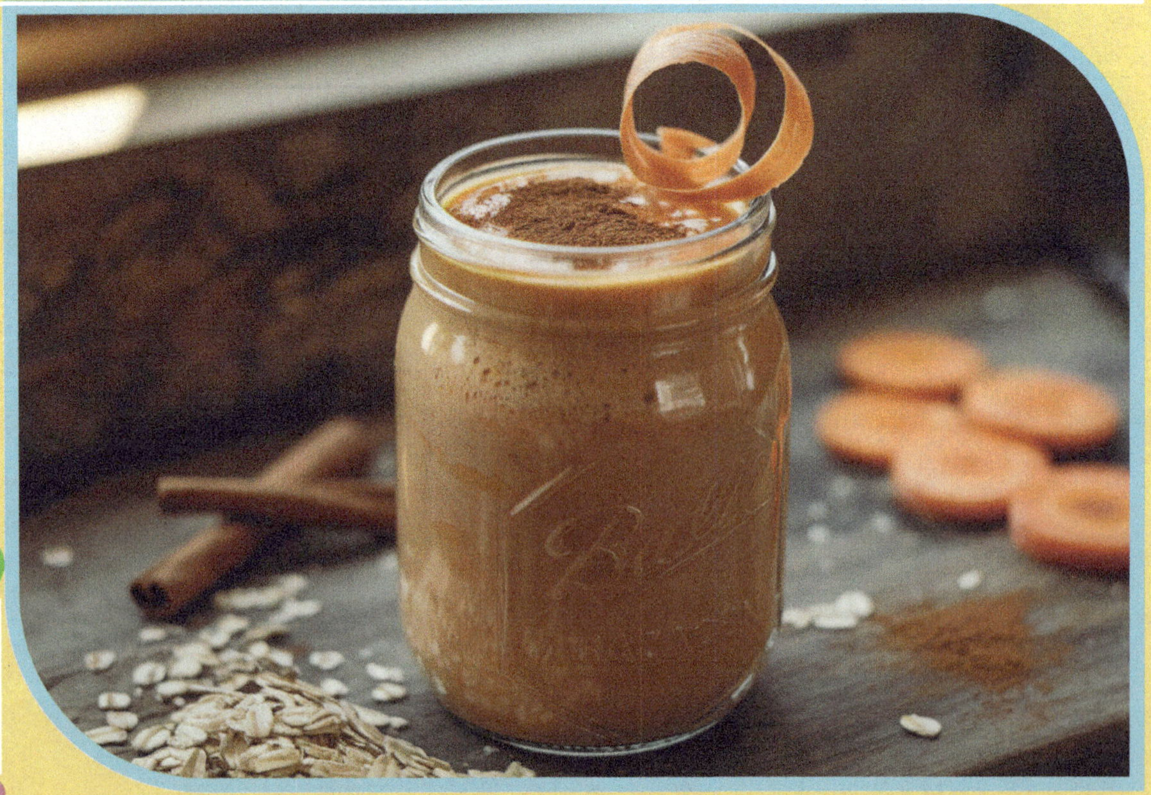

Find this recipe on our website

scan me

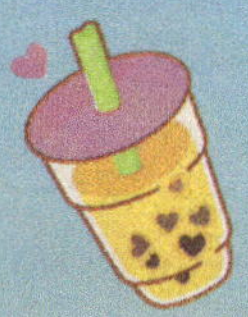

Nutritional & Health Benefits of Carrot Cake Energizer

A Cozy Blend for Afternoon Focus and Balance

Your Carrot Cake Energizer is like dessert with a purpose – rich in fiber, softly spiced, and deeply satisfying.

This smoothie stabilizes afternoon energy while supporting hormone balance and digestion.

It's your perfect pick-me-up when your body needs calm focus, not caffeine crashes.

By Day 12, you've likely noticed improved clarity and lighter digestion – this blend sustains that progress with comfort and care.

Ingredient Power Breakdown

Carrot – High in beta-carotene, which supports skin, immune, and hormone health.

Banana – Offers potassium and vitamin B6 to steady mood and metabolism.

Rolled Oats – Provide soluble fiber to support healthy gut bacteria and prolong fullness.

Cinnamon – Naturally balances blood sugar and reduces mid-afternoon cravings.

Vanilla Extract – Adds warmth and aroma that calms the nervous system.

Honey or Maple Syrup (Optional) – Touch of natural sweetness to sustain steady energy.

Almond or Oat Milk – Calcium-rich base that blends smoothly and supports bone health.

Why It Matters for Women Over 40

This phase of life often brings hormonal fluctuations that affect energy, mood, and metabolism.

The Carrot Cake Energizer helps by:

Supporting estrogen balance through fiber and beta-carotene

Reducing sugar cravings and energy crashes

Promoting better focus with vitamin B6 and cinnamon synergy

Replenishing nutrients needed for natural afternoon vitality

This smoothie delivers comfort, nourishment, and hormonal harmony – all in one glass.

Pro Tip:

Blend with a few ice cubes for a thicker "carrot cake milkshake" texture – a perfect midday treat without the guilt.

🌸 Mind-Body Connection & Lifestyle Insights

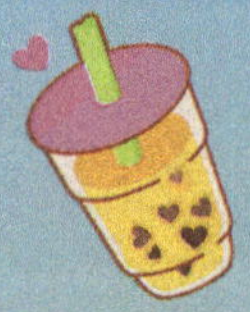

🌤 Today's Focus: Harmony

Balance is the quiet form of strength.

As you sip this creamy orange blend, imagine your body settling into calm energy – not too fast, not too slow – just right.

This is your body learning equilibrium again, one mindful meal at a time.

🧘 Mind-Body Benefits

Cinnamon and vanilla soothe emotional stress and sweet cravings.

Fiber promotes both gut and emotional balance – your gut is your second brain.

Gentle natural sweetness restores calm satisfaction, reducing emotional snacking.

🌿 Mini Habit Challenge

Mid-afternoon, pause for five deep breaths before reaching for your smoothie.

This small act lowers cortisol and improves nutrient absorption – harmony in action.

🖤 Affirmation of the Day

"I move through my day with ease and balance.

My body and mind work together in harmony."

Daily Notes Space:

12

How did this sweet, spiced smoothie affect your energy this afternoon? Note how long it kept you satisfied.

DAY 13 – Power Green Reboot
Early Dinner (before 6 p.m.) : Evening Digestion

- 1 cup fresh spinach leaves
- ½ cup pineapple chunks (fresh or frozen)
- ½ banana
- 1 tablespoon ground flaxseed
- 1 cup unsweetened almond milk (or coconut milk)
- ½ inch piece of fresh ginger (peeled)
- Ice cubes (optional)

- Calories: ~180
- Natural Sugar: ~13 g
- Key Nutrients:
- Vitamin C (pineapple) – boosts immune and collagen production
- Iron & Folate (spinach) – improve circulation and energy levels
- Omega-3s (flaxseed) – support hormone balance and reduce inflammation
- Gingerol (ginger) – aids digestion and calms the stomach
- Fiber: ~5 g

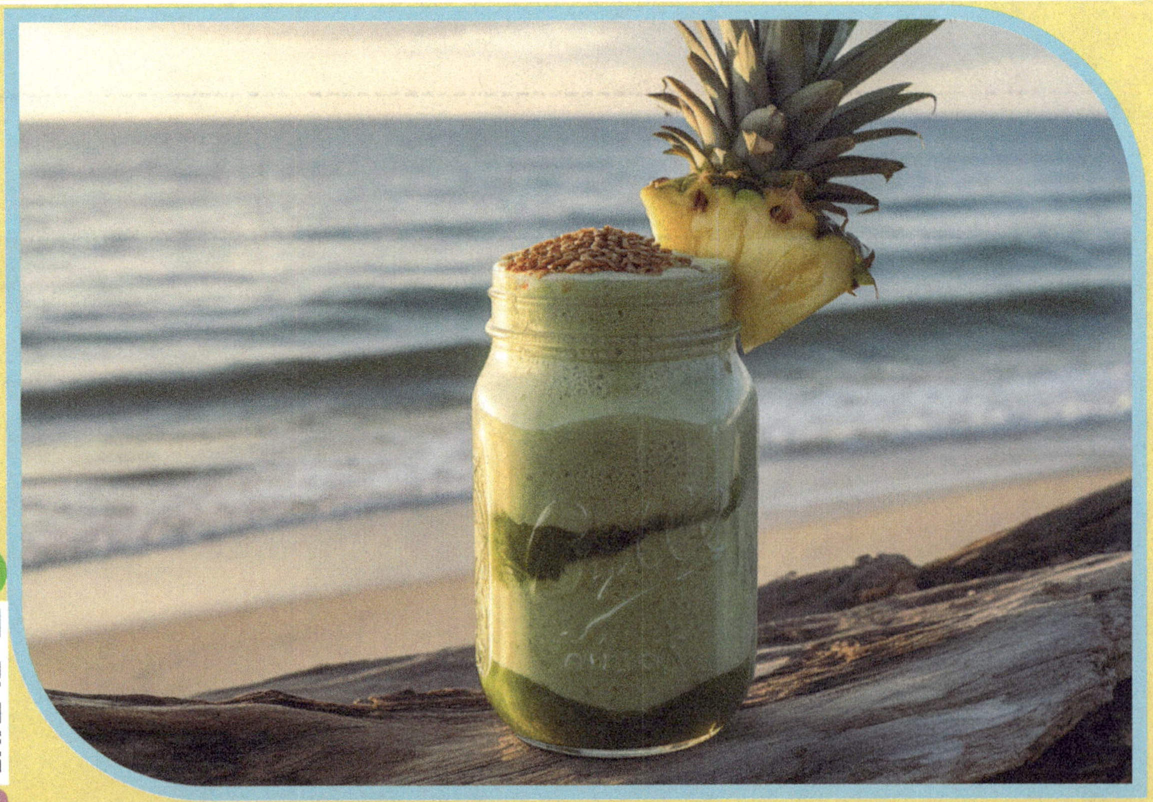

Find this recipe on our website

scan me

🤍 Nutritional & Health Benefits of Power Green Reboot

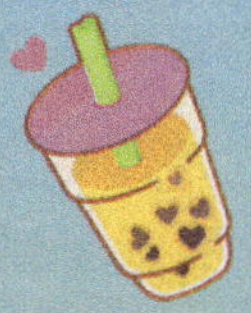

🖤 A Gentle Detox for Hormone Harmony and Calm Digestion

Your Power Green Reboot is a soothing green elixir designed to restore your body's internal rhythm after a full, energizing day.

This blend brings together the cleansing power of greens, the sweetness of pineapple, and the calming touch of ginger – creating a gentle "evening reset" for digestion, hormones, and hydration.

By Day 13, your system is more efficient, your cravings are stabilizing, and your body is naturally seeking balance. This smoothie helps deliver it.

🌿 Ingredient Power Breakdown

Spinach – Iron and folate support oxygen flow, combat fatigue, and aid hormone regulation.

Pineapple – Vitamin C and bromelain promote collagen production and calm inflammation.

Banana – Provides magnesium and potassium for muscle relaxation and nerve balance.

Ground Flaxseed – A source of omega-3s and lignans that help balance estrogen and reduce inflammation.

Ginger – Stimulates digestion and soothes the gut for restful evenings.

Almond or Coconut Milk – Adds creaminess with calcium for bone support and relaxation.

🍀 Why It Matters for Women Over 40

As hormone fluctuations affect digestion, mood, and metabolism, Power Green Reboot provides:

Omega-3s for hormone regulation and anti-inflammatory benefits

Iron and folate to prevent fatigue and support blood health

Ginger and pineapple enzymes for better digestion before sleep

Magnesium and potassium to relax muscles and reduce tension

It's a calm, nutrient-rich way to end your day feeling nourished – not heavy.

✨ Pro Tip:

Blend with a few ice cubes and sip slowly. The natural fiber helps your body absorb nutrients gradually, easing nighttime hunger and supporting gut health.

🌸 Mind-Body Connection & Lifestyle Insights

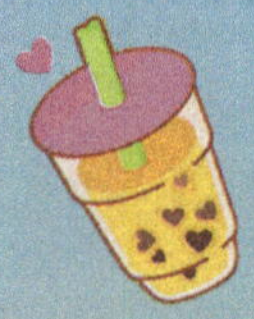

🌙 Today's Focus: Calm & Restore

Evening calm is not a luxury – it's a necessity.

As you enjoy your green smoothie, let your body exhale from the day. This moment of nourishment tells your system: "I'm safe. I can rest."

🧘 Mind-Body Benefits

Calms the nervous system for smoother digestion and better sleep.

Supports hormone balance through stable nutrient intake.

Encourages mindfulness and self-connection during your evening wind-down.

🌿 Mini Habit Challenge

Drink your Power Green Reboot without screens – no phone, no TV, no rush.

Give yourself ten quiet minutes of presence. You'll digest not just food, but the day itself.

💎 Affirmation of the Day

"I nourish my body with calm and care.

Each night, I restore my strength and harmony from within."

Daily Notes Space:

13

How relaxed did you feel after replacing dinner with this smoothie? Did it help your digestion or sleep?

DAY 14 – Weekend Reset Mocha

Breakfast : Mood Lift & Metabolic Kickstart

- 1 small banana
- 1 tablespoon unsweetened cocoa powder
- 1 teaspoon instant coffee or espresso powder (optional for caffeine boost)
- 1 tablespoon almond butter
- 1 cup unsweetened almond milk (or oat milk)
- ½ teaspoon pure vanilla extract
- Ice cubes (optional)

- Calories: ~200
- Natural Sugar: ~10 g
- Key Nutrients:
- Polyphenols (cocoa) – improve mood and support heart health
- Magnesium (almond butter, cocoa) – reduces stress
- Potassium (banana) – balances electrolytes for steady morning energy
- Antioxidants (coffee + cocoa) – protect cells and enhance focus
- Fiber: ~3 g

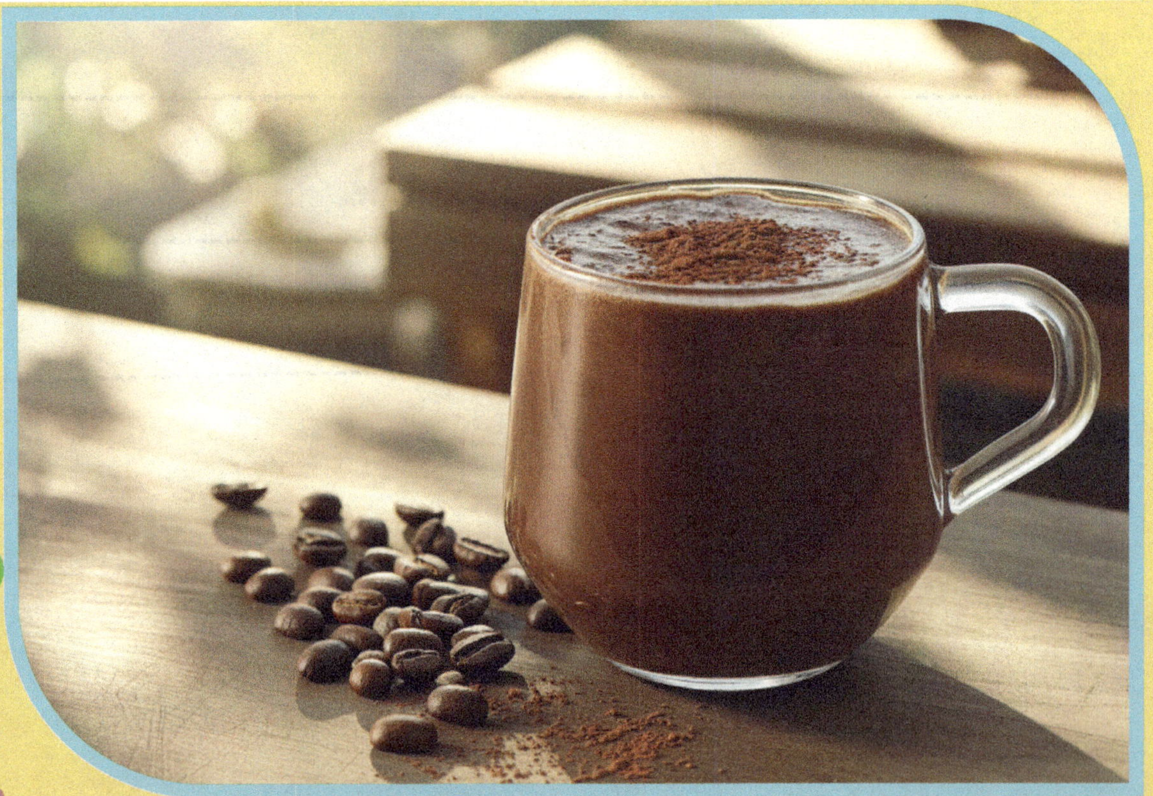

Find this recipe on our website

scan me

Nutritional & Health Benefits of Weekend Reset Mocha

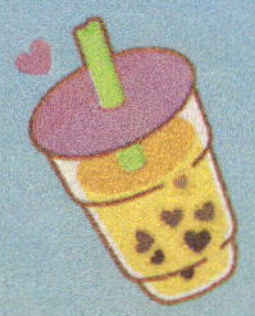

A Cozy Blend for Energy, Mood, and Focus

Your Weekend Reset Mocha is more than a treat – it's a mindful indulgence with benefits. This rich, chocolatey smoothie combines protein, healthy fats, and natural caffeine to recharge your mood and metabolism without relying on sugary lattes or processed snacks. By Day 14, your body has learned consistency. This smoothie gives you permission to relax and enjoy nourishment that feels luxurious yet balanced.

Ingredient Power Breakdown

Cocoa Powder – Packed with polyphenols that boost serotonin, enhance mood, and support heart health.

Instant Coffee or Espresso (Optional) – Adds gentle caffeine for alertness and mental clarity.

Banana – Provides potassium and natural sweetness to prevent energy dips.

Almond Butter – Delivers magnesium and healthy fats to calm stress and sustain energy.

Almond Milk (or Oat Milk) – Smooth, dairy-free base rich in vitamin E for skin protection.

Vanilla Extract – Adds aroma and balance while enhancing antioxidant effects.

Why It Matters for Women Over 40

The Weekend Reset Mocha offers a hormone-friendly caffeine boost – steady, not spiking. It helps by:

Supporting adrenal balance for smoother energy release

Lifting mood naturally through cocoa's serotonin-boosting compounds

Providing magnesium to reduce anxiety and muscle tension

Delivering antioxidants that protect against oxidative stress

This smoothie redefines indulgence: rich, empowering, and restorative.

Pro Tip:

If sensitive to caffeine, replace espresso with roasted chicory or mushroom coffee – same flavor depth, zero jitters.

Mind-Body Connection & Lifestyle Insights

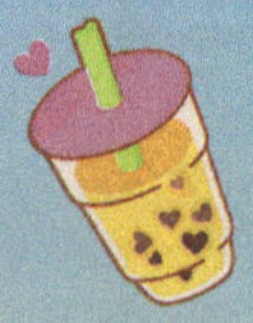

Today's Focus: Reward & Rebalance

You've earned this.

Today is not about restriction – it's about rhythm. Your body thrives when it's allowed both discipline and delight.

As you sip your mocha smoothie, savor the flavor of balance – comfort without compromise.

Mind-Body Benefits

Cocoa and vanilla uplift mood and stimulate dopamine – your "feel good" neurotransmitter.

The ritual of a slow, warm sip invites presence and calm focus.

Pairing caffeine with healthy fats prevents cortisol spikes and emotional crashes.

Mini Habit Challenge

Create a "slow morning" ritual: enjoy your smoothie in silence or with soft music, no screens.

Notice how mindful indulgence restores energy better than multitasking ever could.

Affirmation of the Day

"I honor my body's rhythm.

I can enjoy pleasure and stay balanced – both are part of my wellness."

Daily Notes Space:

14

How did this mocha smoothie affect your morning mood and focus? Track your energy and cravings through the day.

DAY 15 – Metabolism Magic
Lunch : Metabolic Boost & Mental Clarity

- ½ cup brewed green tea (cooled)
- ½ green apple (cored and chopped)
- ½ cup frozen pineapple chunks
- 5–6 fresh mint leaves
- Juice of ½ lime
- ½ teaspoon honey (optional)
- ½ cup cold water or ice cubes

- Calories: ~95
- Natural Sugar: ~11 g
- Key Nutrients:
  - Catechins (green tea) – enhance fat oxidation and mental focus
  - Vitamin C (pineapple, lime) – supports immune and skin health
  - Potassium (apple) – assists fluid balance and circulation
  - Antioxidants (mint) – refresh breath and reduce inflammation
- Fiber: ~3 g

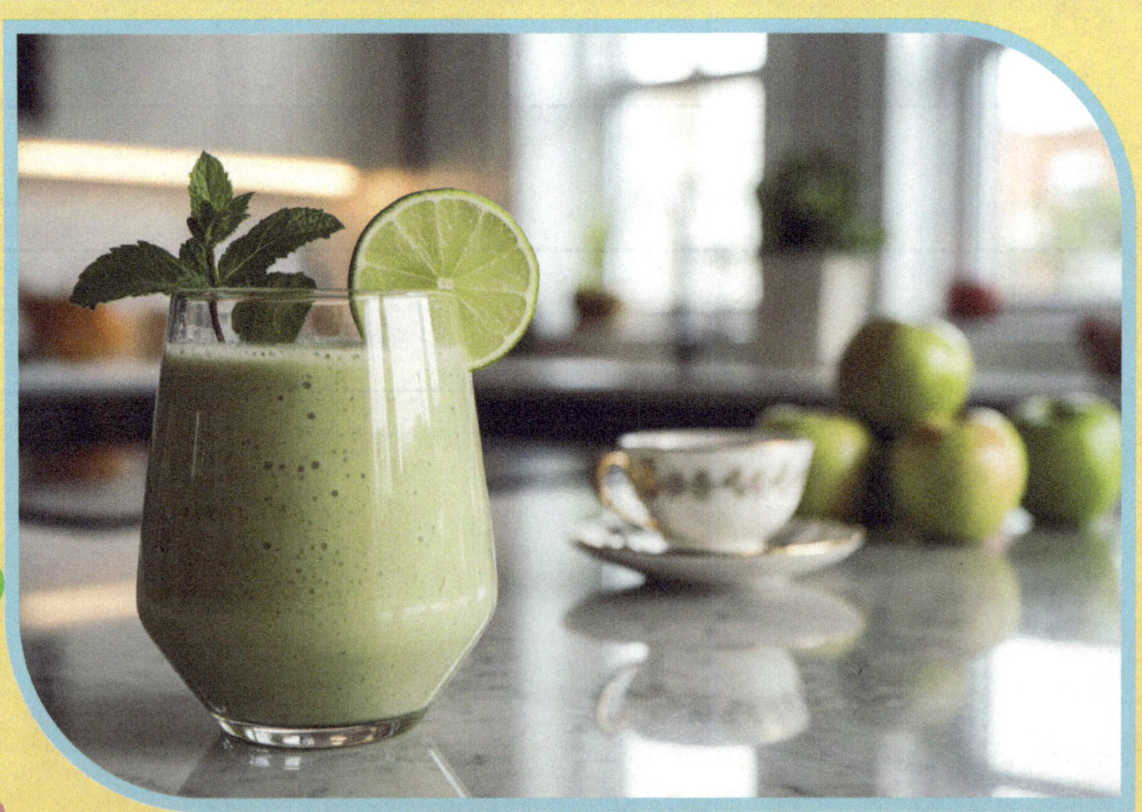

Find this recipe on our website

scan me

🤍 Nutritional & Health Benefits of Metabolism Magic

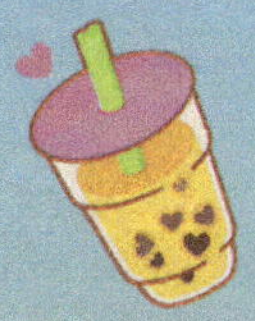

🖤 A Fresh Infusion for Energy and Clarity

Your Metabolism Magic Smoothie is a refreshing midday reboot – hydrating, light, and brimming with natural plant compounds that wake up your metabolism and mind.

By Day 15, your body is running cleaner, your digestion steadier, and your energy levels more predictable. This smoothie enhances that flow by stimulating fat oxidation, calming inflammation, and sharpening mental focus.

🍍 Ingredient Power Breakdown

Green Tea – Contains catechins and mild caffeine that gently boost metabolism and alertness without jitters.

Green Apple – High in fiber and polyphenols that promote fat metabolism and blood sugar control.

Pineapple – Offers bromelain for digestion and vitamin C for collagen production.

Fresh Mint – Soothes the stomach and reduces internal heat.

Lime Juice – Detoxifies the liver and provides antioxidant protection.

Honey (Optional) – A natural energy enhancer rich in trace minerals.

🍀 Why It Matters for Women Over 40

Metabolic rate naturally declines after 40 due to hormonal shifts and stress.

The Metabolism Magic Smoothie helps by:

Gently activating thermogenesis with green tea catechins

Supporting hormone detox through vitamin C and hydration

Enhancing circulation and fat metabolism

Increasing focus and calm energy through polyphenols and mint aroma

This blend is your light lunch magic – a refreshing way to feel sharp, awake, and naturally radiant.

✨ Pro Tip:

For extra fat-burning support, use cold-brewed green tea – the slower extraction maintains antioxidants while lowering bitterness.

Mind-Body Connection & Lifestyle Insights

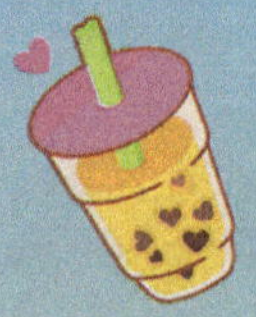

Today's Focus: Mental Clarity

As your body grows stronger, your mind becomes lighter too.
This bright-green blend isn't just for your metabolism – it's a ritual of alert presence.
Sip slowly and feel your awareness expand with every cool, minty note.

Mind-Body Benefits

Promotes clarity through mild caffeine paired with hydration.
Green hues and citrus scents refresh both body and spirit.
Encourages you to pause, breathe, and re-center midday – energy without urgency.

Mini Habit Challenge

Take a five-minute "reset break" today – stretch your body, look outside, breathe deeply, then enjoy your smoothie.
This moment reconnects metabolism and mindfulness.

Affirmation of the Day

"I move with clarity and purpose.
My energy flows easily, my focus is clear, and my body feels alive."

Daily Notes Space:

15 How did this green-tea blend affect your energy and focus this afternoon? Note any changes in mental clarity or hunger levels.

Page intentionally left blank

Thank you so much for reading this book!

We'd Love to hear from You

Review us on Amazon

★★★★★

Scan me

-OR-

Touch or Click here to review

DAY 16 – Omega Balance

Early Dinner (before 6 p.m.) : Hormone Support

- 1 tablespoon ground flaxseed (or chia seeds)
- ½ cup mixed berries (blueberries, raspberries, or strawberries)
- 1 cup fresh spinach leaves
- ½ small banana
- 1 cup unsweetened almond milk (or oat milk)
- ½ teaspoon honey or agave (optional)
- Ice cubes (optional)

- Calories: ~170
- Natural Sugar: ~11 g
- Key Nutrients:
- Omega-3s (flaxseed) – reduce inflammation and support hormone balance
- Antioxidants (berries) – protect against oxidative stress and aging
- Iron & Folate (spinach) – improve circulation and energy
- Fiber (flaxseed, fruit) – aids digestion and satiety
- Fiber: ~6 g

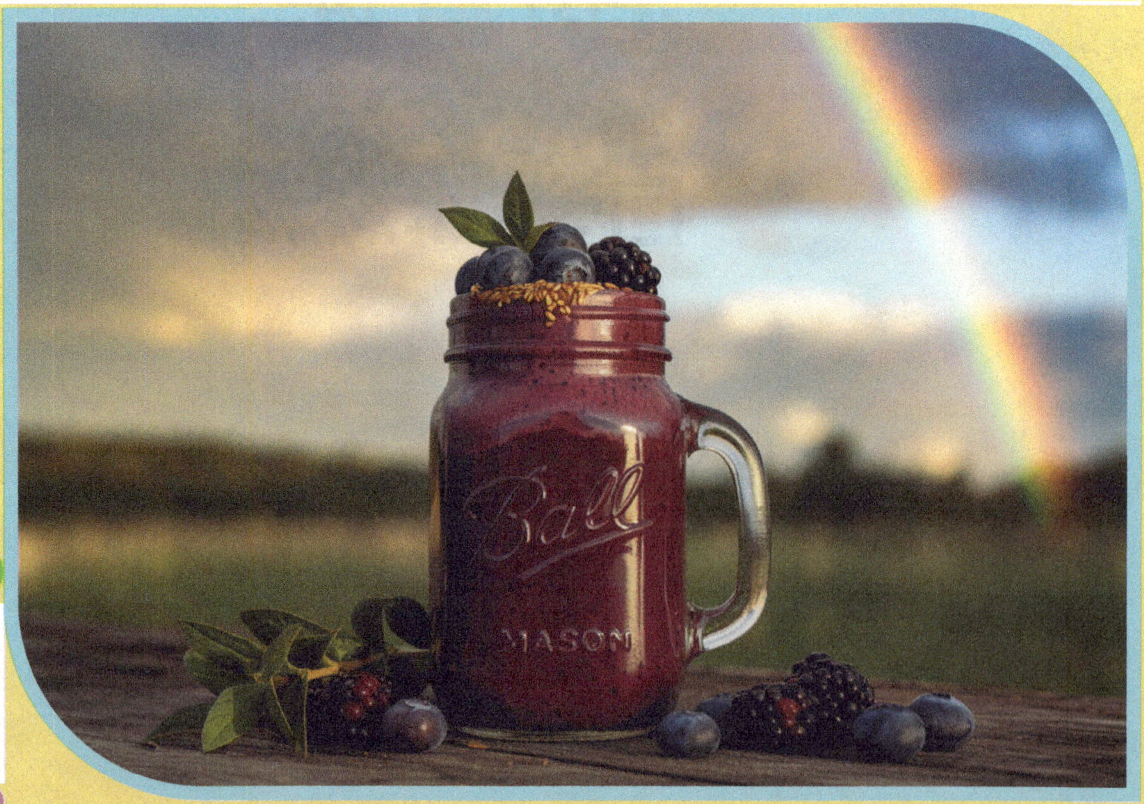

Find this recipe on our website

scan me

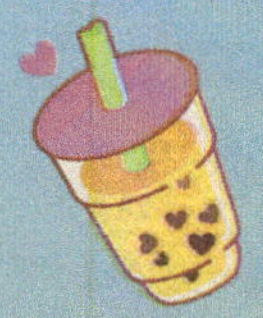

❤ Nutritional & Health Benefits of Omega Balance

🪷 A Rebalancing Blend for Evening Calm and Restoration
Your Omega Balance Smoothie is designed to bring your system back to harmony — smoothing inflammation, restoring calm, and supporting overnight repair.
By Day 16, your metabolism has stabilized, but now your hormones need gentle nourishment to maintain that progress. This omega-rich, antioxidant-packed blend does exactly that.

🌿 Ingredient Power Breakdown
Flaxseed (or Chia Seeds) – Excellent plant-based source of omega-3s that support hormone balance, reduce inflammation, and aid heart health.
Mixed Berries – Loaded with antioxidants and polyphenols that protect against aging and strengthen blood vessels.
Spinach – High in iron and folate to improve circulation and support natural energy.
Banana – Provides potassium and resistant starch to calm the nervous system and ease digestion.
Almond or Oat Milk – Adds creaminess with vitamin E and magnesium for skin and muscle relaxation.
Honey or Agave (Optional) – Natural sweetness that supports serotonin production for a calmer mood.

✿ Why It Matters for Women Over 40
This smoothie supports hormonal and cellular renewal — two essentials for midlife vitality.
It helps by:
Balancing estrogen through plant-based omega-3s and lignans
Reducing chronic inflammation linked to fatigue and skin dullness
Improving blood flow and nutrient delivery to muscles and skin
Promoting restful sleep through magnesium and serotonin synergy
This blend reminds your body that nourishment and peace can coexist beautifully.

✨ Pro Tip:
If drinking before bed, warm the almond milk slightly before blending for a soothing, "nighttime latte" version that enhances absorption and calm.

Mind-Body Connection & Lifestyle Insights

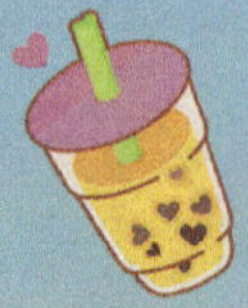

Today's Focus: Inner Balance

Balance is not something you chase – it's something you create through consistency. As you sip this deep-purple smoothie, feel your body settling into its natural rhythm. You're not fighting change – you're flowing with it.

Mind-Body Benefits

Omega-3s regulate mood and reduce cortisol-driven anxiety.
Antioxidants clear oxidative stress that drains emotional energy.
The simple act of evening nourishment signals safety, grounding your system.

Mini Habit Challenge

After your smoothie, dim the lights, stretch gently, and take three deep breaths before bed. Let your body feel the stillness you've earned.

Affirmation of the Day

"I nourish myself with calm and intention.
Balance flows through every part of me – body, mind, and spirit."

Daily Notes Space:

16

Did you feel lighter or calmer after this dinner smoothie? Track any changes in mood, digestion, or sleep quality.

DAY 17 – Vanilla Chia Recovery

Breakfast : Muscle Recovery & Morning Calm

- 1 tablespoon chia seeds
- 1 small banana
- 1 cup unsweetened almond milk (or oat milk)
- ½ teaspoon pure vanilla extract
- ½ teaspoon cinnamon (optional)
- 1 teaspoon honey or maple syrup (optional)
- Ice cubes (optional)

- Calories: ~190
- Natural Sugar: ~10 g
- Key Nutrients:
- Omega-3s (chia seeds) – reduce inflammation and aid tissue recovery
- Potassium (banana) – supports muscle repair and hydration
- Calcium (almond milk) – strengthens bones and balances nerves
- Magnesium (chia, banana) – relaxes muscles and promotes steady energy
- Fiber: ~6 g

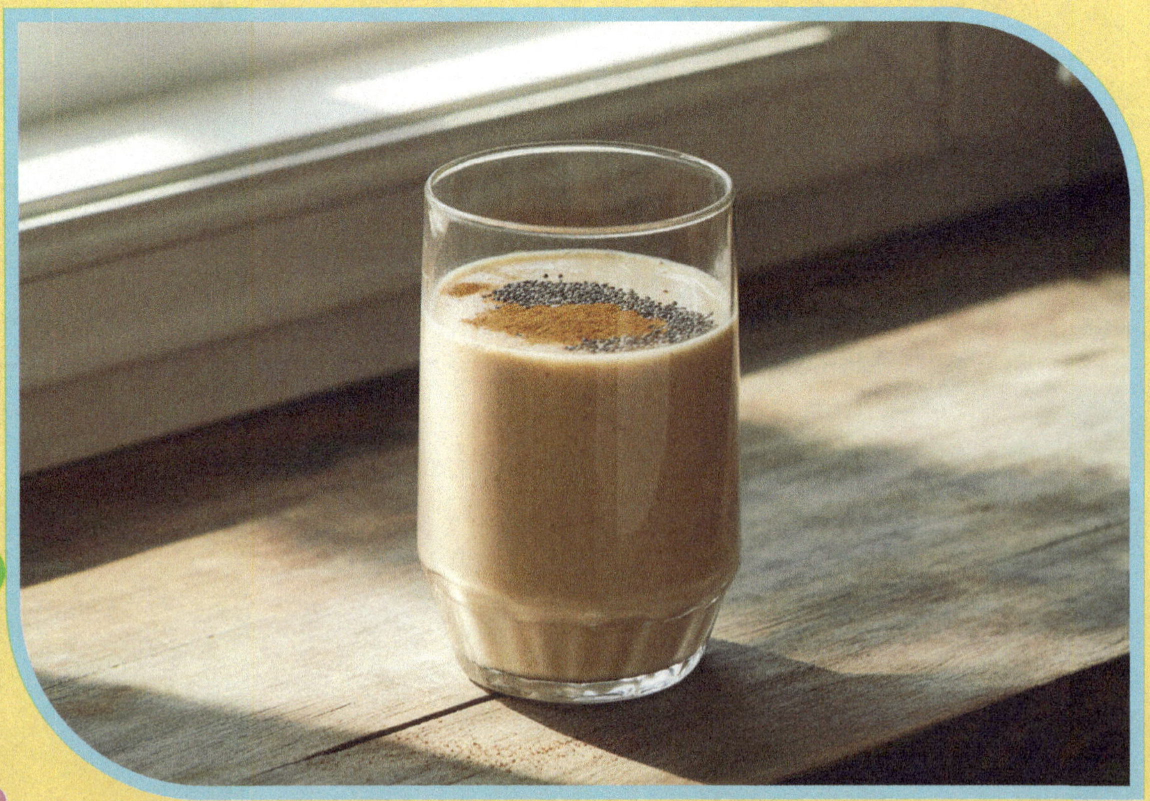

Find this recipe on our website

scan me

🌿 Nutritional & Health Benefits of Vanilla Chia Recovery

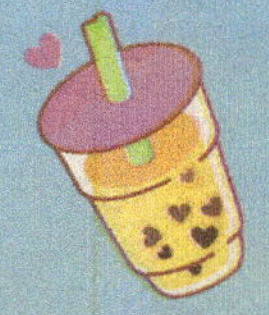

🖤 A Gentle Rebuilder for Strength and Serenity

Your Vanilla Chia Recovery Smoothie is the calm after the storm — creamy, light, and deeply satisfying.

This blend replenishes essential minerals, repairs muscles, and restores inner calm after physical or emotional exertion. It's the perfect way to wake up your body with grace, not rush.

By Day 17, your system is balanced and responsive. This smoothie nurtures that stability with protein, fiber, and magnesium to keep you grounded and energized throughout the morning.

🍌 Ingredient Power Breakdown

Chia Seeds – Rich in omega-3s, fiber, and plant protein that promote tissue recovery and hormone balance.

Banana – Provides potassium and magnesium for muscle relaxation and hydration.

Almond or Oat Milk – Adds calcium for bone health and vitamin E for skin protection.

Vanilla Extract – Naturally soothing aroma that reduces stress and enhances flavor.

Cinnamon (Optional) – Balances blood sugar and supports warm, stable energy.

Honey or Maple Syrup (Optional) – Adds light sweetness and trace antioxidants.

🌸 Why It Matters for Women Over 40

This smoothie helps women rebuild strength and balance hormones after periods of stress or fatigue.

It supports:

Muscle and tissue repair with amino acids and magnesium

Hormonal equilibrium through steady omega-3 intake

Gut regularity and natural detoxification via soluble fiber

Calm, focused mornings without caffeine dependence

This is your gentle reset smoothie — nourishing without heaviness, calming without slowing you down.

✨ Pro Tip:

Blend and let rest 3–5 minutes before drinking. This allows chia to expand — improving digestion, satiety, and texture.

Mind-Body Connection & Lifestyle Insights

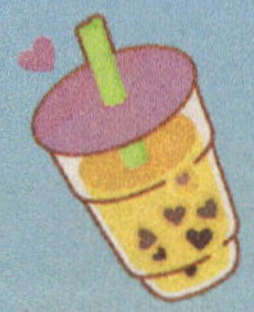

Today's Focus: Recovery & Renewal

Recovery is not weakness – it's where strength is rebuilt.

As you sip this smooth, vanilla-scented blend, imagine each cell being restored, hydrated, and rebalanced.

This moment isn't about doing – it's about allowing.

Mind-Body Benefits

Omega-3s soothe the nervous system, easing stress and anxiety.

Steady glucose release supports mood stability and focus.

The act of pausing – blending, waiting, sipping – teaches mindful patience.

Mini Habit Challenge

Before your smoothie, stretch for 3 minutes.

Feel your breath expand into every muscle you're nourishing.

Recovery is movement in slow motion.

Affirmation of the Day

"I restore myself with calm and care.

My energy rebuilds gently and flows with purpose."

Daily Notes Space:

17

Did you notice better focus or reduced fatigue after this breakfast smoothie? Record how your body and mind felt today.

DAY 18 – Digestive Harmony

Lunch : Gut Health & Digestive Balance

- ½ cup ripe papaya (peeled, seeded, and cubed)
- ½ banana
- ¼ cup plain Greek yogurt (unsweetened)
- ½ inch piece fresh ginger (peeled)
- 1 teaspoon honey (optional)
- ¾ cup unsweetened almond milk (or coconut milk)
- Ice cubes (optional)

- Calories: ~160
- Natural Sugar: ~12 g
- Key Nutrients:
- Digestive enzymes (papaya) – assist in breaking down proteins and reducing bloating
- Probiotics (Greek yogurt) – promote gut flora balance and immunity
- Vitamin C (papaya, banana) – aids tissue repair and radiant skin
- Gingerol (ginger) – reduces gut inflammation and nausea
- Fiber: ~3 g

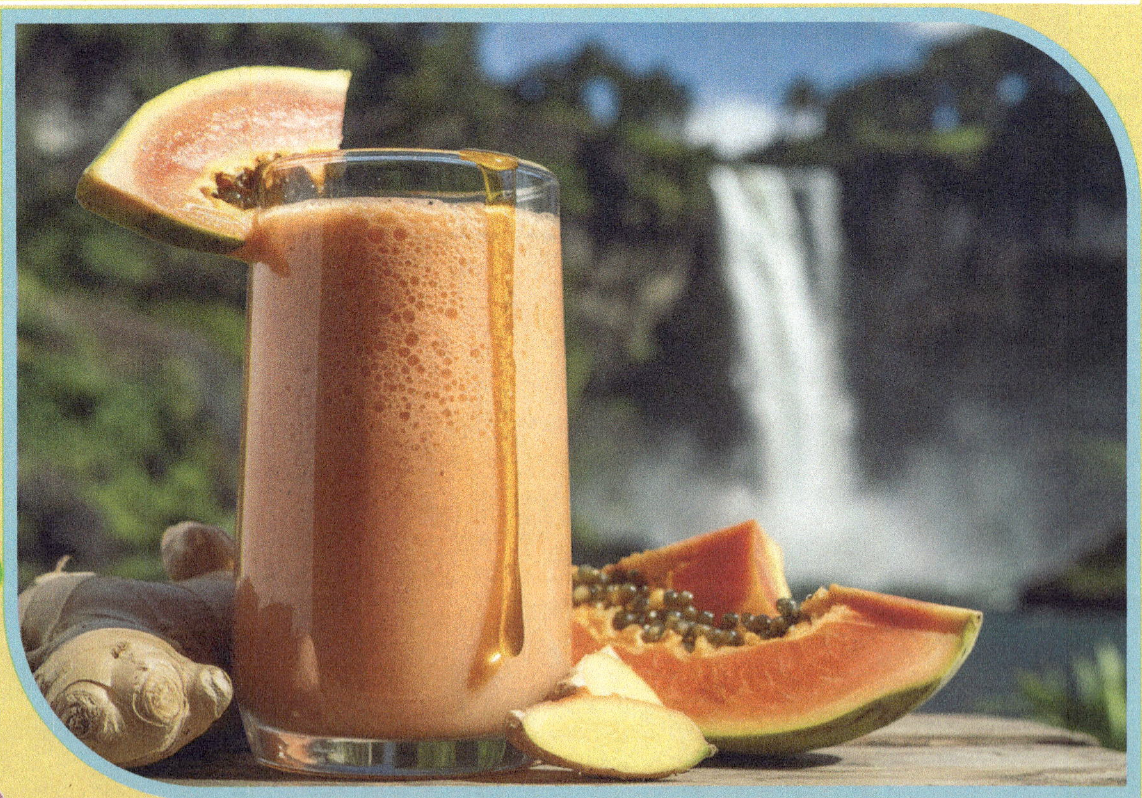

Find this recipe on our website

scan me

🧘 Nutritional & Health Benefits of Digestive Harmony

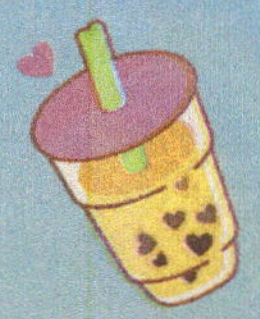

🍎 A Gentle Reset for Gut and Glow

Your Digestive Harmony Smoothie is a soft, creamy blend that works like a wellness massage for your digestive system.

Papaya's natural enzymes soothe the stomach, while probiotics and ginger reduce inflammation and promote regularity.

By Day 18, your body is in a beautiful state of equilibrium – this smoothie keeps your gut balanced, your skin glowing, and your energy smooth.

🌿 Ingredient Power Breakdown

Papaya – Contains papain, a natural digestive enzyme that helps break down protein and reduce bloating.

Banana – Offers prebiotic fiber to feed healthy gut bacteria and restore calm to the digestive tract.

Greek Yogurt – Provides probiotics for a balanced microbiome and stronger immunity.

Ginger – Eases nausea, stimulates digestion, and soothes intestinal inflammation.

Honey (Optional) – Adds gentle sweetness and antibacterial benefits.

Almond or Coconut Milk – Light, soothing base that hydrates and supports nutrient absorption.

🌸 Why It Matters for Women Over 40

A healthy gut is the foundation of hormone balance, energy, and mood.

The Digestive Harmony Smoothie supports this by:

Restoring gut flora disrupted by stress or poor diet

Reducing bloating and supporting regular digestion

Improving nutrient absorption for clearer skin and better energy

Calming inflammation that affects mood and immunity

This smoothie is your inner harmony in a glass – gentle, glowing, and grounded.

✨ Pro Tip:

For even better digestion, drink this smoothie slowly and slightly chilled. The enzymes in papaya and probiotics in yogurt work best when not exposed to high temperatures.

Mind-Body Connection & Lifestyle Insights

Today's Focus: Inner Ease

When your gut feels good, your whole world feels lighter.

As you sip this tropical, soothing blend, think of digestion as more than a process – it's your body's conversation with itself.

Harmony begins here.

Mind-Body Benefits

Supports emotional calm through gut-brain connection.

Reduces stress by lowering inflammation in the digestive tract.

Encourages patience and presence through mindful nourishment.

Mini Habit Challenge

Before drinking, take a few deep breaths and relax your abdomen.

This simple act activates the parasympathetic ("rest and digest") system, helping your body absorb every nutrient more effectively.

Affirmation of the Day

"I am at peace with my body.

My digestion flows smoothly, and balance radiates from within."

Daily Notes Space:

18

Did your stomach feel lighter after this smoothie? Track any changes in digestion, bloating, or comfort through the afternoon.

DAY 19 – Chocolate Mood Lift

Early Dinner (before 6 p.m.) : Mood Boost & Stress Relief

- 1 tablespoon unsweetened cocoa powder
- 1 tablespoon almond butter
- ½ frozen banana
- 1 teaspoon honey or maple syrup (optional)
- 1 cup unsweetened almond milk (or oat milk)
- ½ teaspoon cinnamon (optional)
- Ice cubes (optional)

- Calories: ~210
- Natural Sugar: ~9 g
- Key Nutrients:
- Theobromine (cocoa) – boosts mood and focus naturally
- Healthy fats (almond butter) – support hormones and satiety
- Magnesium (cocoa, almonds) – eases stress and muscle tension
- Potassium (banana) – maintains hydration and nerve balance
- Fiber: ~4 g

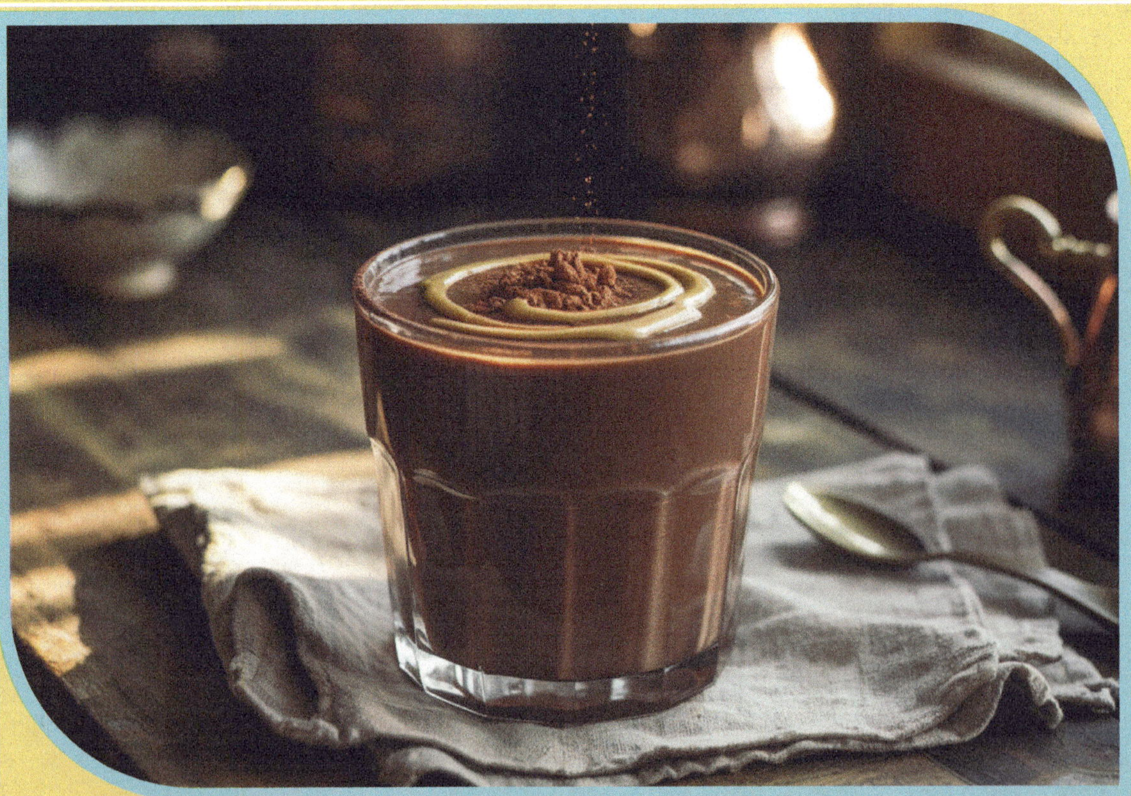

Find this recipe on our website

scan me

Nutritional & Health Benefits of Chocolate Mood Lift

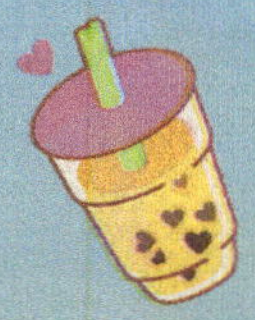

A Comforting Blend for Calm and Happiness

Your Chocolate Mood Lift Smoothie is proof that healthy can feel heavenly.

This rich, creamy blend delivers the taste of dessert with the chemistry of calm – pairing magnesium-rich cocoa and healthy fats to lift your mood, relax your body, and ease evening cravings.

By Day 19, your energy has balanced, your cravings are fewer, and your body is more attuned to nourishment over impulse. This smoothie celebrates that progress – comforting yet empowering.

Ingredient Power Breakdown

Cocoa Powder – Packed with theobromine and magnesium to elevate mood, focus, and relaxation.

Almond Butter – Provides monounsaturated fats and vitamin E for hormonal support and lasting fullness.

Banana – Adds potassium and serotonin precursors for natural happiness and calm.

Cinnamon (Optional) – Enhances circulation and helps regulate cortisol (your stress hormone).

Almond or Oat Milk – Smooth, dairy-free base for skin-friendly vitamin E.

Why It Matters for Women Over 40

Fluctuating estrogen levels can affect serotonin, mood, and stress tolerance.

The Chocolate Mood Lift Smoothie helps by:

Boosting serotonin and dopamine naturally through cocoa and banana

Providing magnesium to reduce anxiety, cramps, and tension

Supporting hormone balance with vitamin E and omega-rich fats

Offering guilt-free indulgence that satisfies cravings without sugar crashes

This is emotional self-care disguised as chocolate bliss.

Pro Tip:

For a richer flavor and extra protein, blend in half a scoop of chocolate or vanilla protein powder – it transforms your smoothie into a "fit dessert."

Mind-Body Connection & Lifestyle Insights

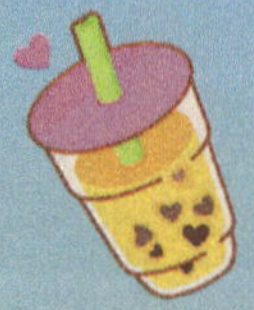

Today's Focus: Joy & Release

You've done the work – now it's time to enjoy the reward.
As you sip this velvety smoothie, let go of the day's weight.
Pleasure isn't the opposite of discipline – it's part of the balance that keeps you thriving.

Mind-Body Benefits

Cocoa's natural theobromine gently stimulates happiness and focus.
Healthy fats signal safety, lowering stress-driven hunger.
The sensory richness of chocolate activates calm and satisfaction centers in the brain.

Mini Habit Challenge

Sip your smoothie slowly and think of one thing you're grateful for today.
Gratitude and chocolate – two proven ways to lift the spirit naturally.

Affirmation of the Day

"I deserve joy, calm, and sweetness.
My choices nourish both my body and my happiness."

Daily Notes Space:

19

Did this smoothie help you unwind or reduce stress this evening? Record your energy and mood before bedtime.

DAY 20 – Golden Glow Tonic

Breakfast : Joint Support & Radiant Skin

- 1 cup fresh or frozen pineapple chunks
- ½ banana
- ½ teaspoon ground turmeric (or ½ inch fresh turmeric root, peeled)
- ½ teaspoon grated fresh ginger
- 1 cup light coconut milk (or unsweetened almond milk)
- 1 teaspoon honey or maple syrup (optional)
- Pinch of black pepper (enhances turmeric absorption)
- Ice cubes (optional)

- Calories: ~180
- Natural Sugar: ~13 g
- Key Nutrients:
- Curcumin (turmeric) – reduces inflammation and supports joint health
- Bromelain (pineapple) – aids digestion and immune defense
- Medium-chain fats (coconut milk) – fuel steady energy and brain focus
- Vitamin C (pineapple, banana) – brightens skin and supports collagen
- Fiber: ~3 g

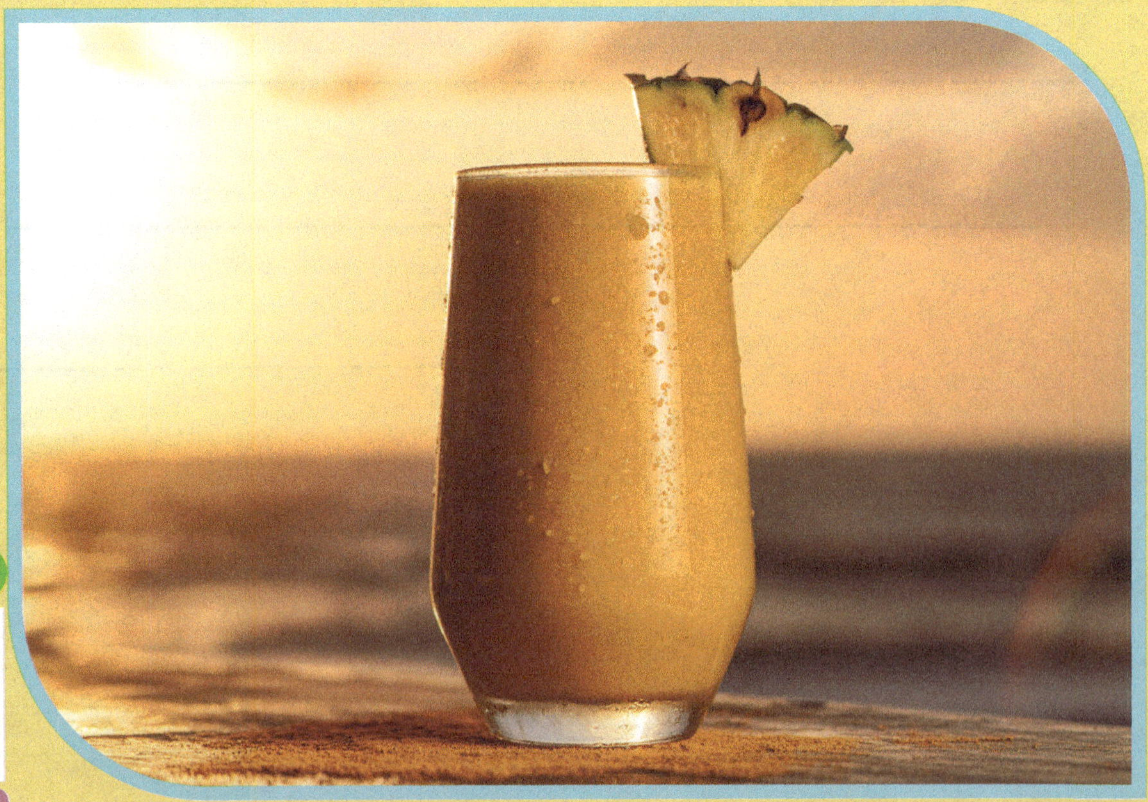

Find this recipe on our website

scan me

Nutritional & Health Benefits of Golden Glow Tonic

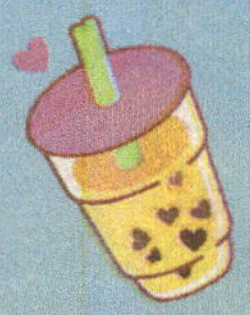

✨ A Bright Blend for Radiance and Renewal

Your Golden Glow Tonic is sunshine in a glass — golden, creamy, and powerfully restorative. This tropical anti-inflammatory blend combines turmeric, pineapple, and coconut to help joints move freely, skin shine naturally, and your energy rise smoothly.

By Day 20, your body has shed sluggishness and reset its natural rhythm. This blend supports that final transformation — vibrant, light, and full of glow.

🍍 Ingredient Power Breakdown

Turmeric – Rich in curcumin, nature's anti-inflammatory compound that supports joint comfort and skin repair.

Pineapple – Contains bromelain, an enzyme that aids digestion and boosts immune defense.

Banana – Adds potassium for hydration and muscle recovery.

Coconut Milk – Delivers medium-chain fatty acids for sustained energy and mental focus.

Ginger – Enhances circulation and promotes detoxification through gentle warmth.

Honey or Maple Syrup (Optional) – A natural energizer that harmonizes turmeric's earthy flavor.

Black Pepper – Boosts curcumin absorption for greater healing power.

Why It Matters for Women Over 40

The Golden Glow Tonic supports long-term vitality by addressing inflammation — the root of fatigue, stiffness, and dull skin.

It helps by:

Reducing joint pain and muscle soreness

Supporting collagen synthesis and skin elasticity

Enhancing liver detox and digestive clarity

Stabilizing energy through healthy fats and antioxidants

This is your daily anti-aging ritual — radiant, energizing, and deeply restorative.

✨ Pro Tip:

Add a pinch of cinnamon or cardamom for warmth and deeper flavor. These spices complement turmeric beautifully and support additional antioxidant benefits.

🌼 Mind-Body Connection & Lifestyle Insights

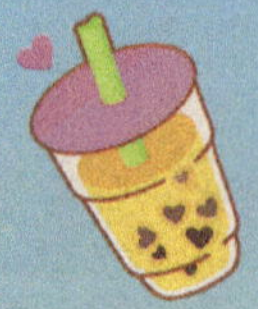

🌅 Today's Focus: Vitality & Radiance

You've nearly completed your 21-day journey – and it shows.

As you sip your golden smoothie, notice how your skin feels smoother, your energy lighter, your confidence brighter.

This isn't just a glow on the outside – it's balance shining from within.

🧘‍♀️ Mind-Body Benefits

Turmeric and ginger reduce inflammation that clouds both body and mood.

The golden color stimulates optimism and creativity.

Mindful sipping helps you connect with gratitude and presence.

✨ Mini Habit Challenge

Stand in natural light as you drink your smoothie.

Breathe in the sunlight, feel it on your skin, and repeat: "I am vibrant. I am renewed."

💛 Affirmation of the Day

"I radiate health, strength, and warmth.

My glow comes from harmony, nourishment, and joy."

Daily Notes Space:

20

Did this golden smoothie help ease stiffness or brighten your mood? Note how your energy and focus felt through the morning.

DAY 21 – Queen's Finale Smoothie

Lunch : Full-Body Renewal & Long-Term Balance

- ½ cup mixed berries (blueberries, strawberries, raspberries)
- ½ cup baby spinach leaves
- ½ banana
- 1 tablespoon mixed seeds (chia, flax, or sunflower)
- 1 cup unsweetened almond milk (or oat milk)
- ½ teaspoon pure vanilla extract
- Ice cubes (optional)

- Calories: ~190
- Natural Sugar: ~11 g
- Key Nutrients:
- Antioxidants (berries, spinach) – protect cells and promote longevity
- Omega-3s & healthy fats (seed blend) – stabilize hormones and support brain health
- Vitamin C (berries) – enhances collagen and immune strength
- Iron & Folate (spinach) – restore post-detox vitality
- Fiber: ~6 g

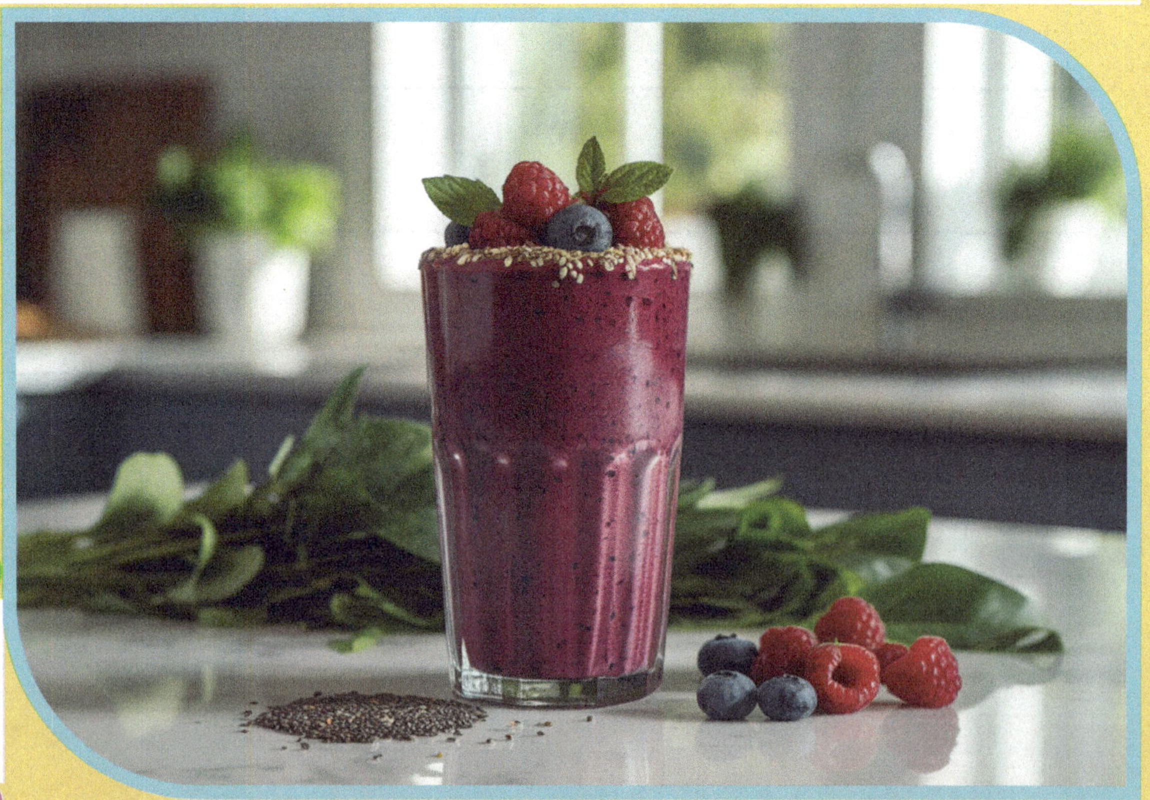

Find this recipe on our website

scan me

👑 Nutritional & Health Benefits of Queen's Finale Smoothie

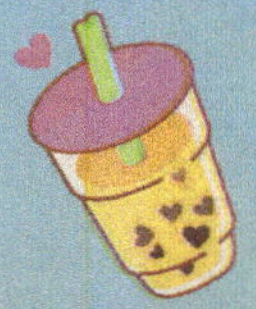

🖤 A Regal Blend for Renewal & Longevity

Your Queen's Finale Smoothie crowns your 21-day transformation with balance, brilliance, and strength.

This rich, jewel-toned blend celebrates everything you've built – resilience, nourishment, and self-trust.

It's a nutrient powerhouse that restores vitality, seals in your glow, and keeps your momentum alive long after the program ends.

By Day 21, your digestion is smoother, your energy steadier, and your body tuned to wellness. This smoothie nourishes your new rhythm and helps you stay aligned with the healthy lifestyle you've created.

🍓 Ingredient Power Breakdown

Mixed Berries – Overflowing with antioxidants that protect cells, support heart health, and encourage youthful skin.

Spinach – Provides iron and folate for sustained energy and post-detox recovery.

Banana – Adds potassium to maintain hydration and balance nerve function.

Mixed Seeds (Chia, Flax, Sunflower) – Deliver omega-3s and vitamin E for hormone balance, brain clarity, and glowing skin.

Vanilla Extract – Brings warmth and comfort to mark the completion of your journey.

Almond or Oat Milk – A light, calcium-rich base that supports bone strength and smooth texture.

🌸 Why It Matters for Women Over 40

The Queen's Finale Smoothie anchors the results you've earned – steady metabolism, glowing skin, and inner harmony.

It helps by:

Restoring antioxidants lost through stress and environmental toxins

Supporting hormone balance with plant-based fats and minerals

Enhancing collagen and immune strength through vitamin C

Promoting long-term energy and cellular renewal

This final blend is not the end – it's the beginning of your new baseline for wellness.

✨ Pro Tip:

Freeze extra berries in small bags so you can keep making this smoothie once a week. It's the easiest way to sustain your post-detox vitality.

🌸 Mind-Body Connection & Lifestyle Insights

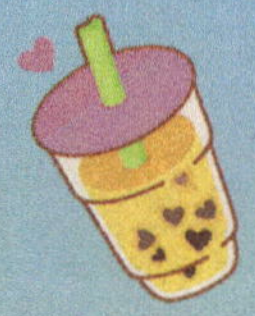

🕊 Today's Focus: Celebration & Continuation

You've shown up for 21 days – not with perfection, but with purpose.
As you sip this vibrant, life-filled smoothie, reflect on how far you've come.
You didn't just finish a program – you rewrote your relationship with food, energy, and self-care.
This moment is your coronation – you are the Queen of your own wellness journey. 👑

🧘🧠 Mind-Body Benefits

Antioxidants protect your body while gratitude protects your mind.
Balanced fats and greens stabilize hormones that nurture long-term calm.
Celebration itself releases endorphins – the true "glow hormone."

✨ Mini Habit Challenge

Write a short "Royal Ritual List" – 3 small habits you'll keep after the detox (e.g., one smoothie a day, nightly stretch, digital-free mornings).
Transformation lasts when it's crowned with consistency.

💖 Affirmation of the Day

"I am radiant, renewed, and powerful.
This isn't the end of my journey – it's my new beginning."

Daily Notes Space:

21

Congratulations! You've completed your 21-day detox journey. Note how your body feels, your favorite smoothies, and any lifestyle changes you plan to keep.

Page intentionally left blank

Thank you so much for reading this book!

We'd Love to hear from You

Review us on Amazon

★★★★★

Scan me

-OR-

Touch or Click here to review

Made in the USA
Monee, IL
02 November 2026

67387003R00059